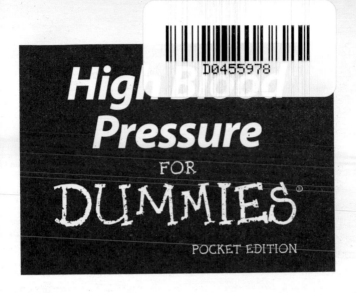

High Blood Pressure

FOR

DUMMIES

POCKET EDITION

by Alan L. Rubin, MD

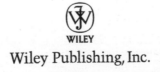

WILEY

Wiley Publishing, Inc.

High Blood Pressure For Dummies,® Pocket Edition

Published by
Wiley Publishing, Inc.
111 River St.
Hoboken, NJ 07030-5774
www.wiley.com

For general information on our other products and services, please contact our Customer Care Department within the U.S. at 877-762-2974, outside the U.S. at 317-572-3993, or fax 317-572-4002. For technical support, please visit www.wiley.com/techsupport.

Wiley also publishes its books in a variety of electronic formats and by print-on-demand. Some content that appears in standard print versions of this book may not be available in other formats. For more information about Wiley products, visit us at www.wiley.com.

ISBN: 978-0-470-91591-2

Manufactured in the United States of America

10 9 8 7 6 5 4 3 2

Publisher's Acknowledgements

Project Editor: Traci Cumbay
Composition Services: Indianapolis Composition Services Department
Cover Photo: © iStockphoto.com/Emilia Stasiak

WILEY

Table of Contents

Chapter 8: Ten Myths about High Blood Pressure...123

Introduction

● ●

*W*hen I was growing up, my mother often used the pressure cooker to make dinner in a hurry. The idea was that if you cooked food at higher pressures, the food would get done faster. High blood pressure in people is like that. If you permit yourself to have high blood pressure, you'll get done faster. What do I mean by *done?* I am talking about all the medical complications, such as heart attack, stroke, and kidney failure, as well as the shortened life span of people with poorly treated or untreated high blood pressure.

High blood pressure, or *hypertension;* as doctors like to call it, affects more than 50 million adults in the United States and between 15 and 25 percent of the rest of the world according to the World Health Organization.

Like diabetes, high blood pressure is a lifestyle disease. It tends to occur in more affluent nations where food is plentiful and hard manual labor is done less often. This is both a problem and a challenge. On the one hand, affluent societies don't want to give up their benefits. On the other, the more fortunate want to enjoy their blessings without destroying themselves.

I always like to have a bottom line in my books, and this one is no exception. The bottom line is that you never have to suffer any of the consequences of high blood pressure. You have it within your brain and your body to prevent it or successfully treat high blood pressure should you discover that you have it. Imagine if all the people with high blood pressure heeded this advice and got theirs under control. About 250,000 lives a year would be saved, not to mention a much larger number who suffer but don't die. And that's in the United States alone.

If you read any of my previous books, *Diabetes For Dummies, Diabetes Cookbook For Dummies,* or *Thyroid For Dummies,* you know that I use humor to get my point across, a technique that characterizes the *For Dummies* series. I want to emphasize that I'm not trying to trivialize anyone's suffering by being comic about it. Humor has healing properties. A positive attitude is far more conducive to a positive outcome than is a negative attitude.

About This Book

No one expects that you'll read this book from cover to cover. You don't have to skip back to Chapter 2 to understand Chapter 7. You don't have to start at the beginning to understand the end. It's not a novel, after all, but a tool to help you manage your high blood pressure. (Though some people may think of high blood pressure as a villain.)

Conventions Used in This Book

As much as I would love to use all nonscientific terms in this book, if I do so, you and your doctor will be speaking two different languages. Therefore, I use the scientific term, but I explain it with simple language the first time you see it.

As for using the term *high blood pressure* or the word *hypertension,* in this case and in all cases, I use the simpler term — high blood pressure. This seems to be the trend, and I think it's a good trend so long as the information that the term provides is accurate and comprehensive.

What You Don't Have to Read

Throughout the book, shaded areas (called sidebars) contain material that's interesting but not essential to your understanding. If you don't care to go so deeply into a subject, skip the sidebars. You'll understand everything else.

Foolish Assumptions

This book makes no assumptions about what you know. All new terms are explained. If you already know a great deal, you'll find new information that adds to your knowledge. Key points are always marked clearly for you. You probably fall into one of the following categories:

- ✔ You've been diagnosed with high blood pressure but haven't started treatment.

- ✔ You're being treated for high blood pressure but aren't happy with the results.

- ✔ You have a close friend or family member with high blood pressure.

Icons Used in This Book

Books in the *For Dummies* series feature icons, which direct you toward information that may be of particular interest or importance. Here's an explanation of what each icon in this book signifies:

I define medical terms where you see this icon.

 When you see this icon, it means the information is essential. You want to be sure you understand it.

 When you find this alongside some information, it's time to dial the doctor for help.

 This icon points out important information that can save you time and energy.

 This icon warns against potential problems (for example if you mix the wrong drugs).

Where to Go From Here

Where you go from here depends on your needs. You're welcome to read straight through or to skip around the book, reading whatever interests you or addresses your questions.

If you want even more information on high blood pressure, from details about medications to more about managing high blood pressure through lifestyle changes, check out the full-size version of *High Blood Pressure For Dummies* (Wiley). Simply head to your local bookseller or go to www.dummies.com.

As my mother used to say when she gave me a present, use this book in good health.

Chapter 1

Getting Acquainted with High Blood Pressure

● ●

In This Chapter

▶ Moving the blood through the cardiovascular system

▶ Defining what determines high blood pressure and its consequences

▶ Getting a diagnosis

▶ Preventing high blood pressure and looking at treatment options

● ●

If you have high blood pressure, you're in good (if not terribly healthy) company. Fifty million Americans (one in four adults) have high blood pressure. A list of the people in this country with high blood pressure would read like a Who's Who. The problem is that without proper treatment many of those people will be on a list of Who Was Who sooner than they may want. Don't let yourself or a loved one get on the Who Was Who list without a fight.

You can do so much about high blood pressure. First, you can prevent it. If your blood pressure is already high, you can control it. But before you can do these things, you need to know what high blood pressure is and how you measure it. Then understanding what's known about how high blood pressure occurs and how it's treated is important.

This book is your blood pressure companion. It provides you with a solid understanding of your blood pressure: how it affects your body — organ by organ, who is at risk, how you can prevent it, and how you can treat high blood pressure after it's properly diagnosed. Lastly, you'll find out about myths associated with high blood pressure.

As you'll discover, a few simple alterations to your lifestyle can prevent high blood pressure. My hope is that as you read the information in this book, you'll be spurred to make healthy changes, not just now but continuing into the future. High blood pressure is a chronic disease. You may lower your blood pressure in the short term, but the goal is long-term control to prevent other medical consequences (which I discuss in Chapter 3).

Take charge of your blood pressure now, and you won't have the fate of a health food store owner who posted a sign that read, "Closed due to illness."

Understanding Your Cardiovascular System

To understand how elevated blood pressure affects your overall health, it's important to understand what makes Thumper tick — well, pump. Your cardiovascular system — your heart, arteries, veins capillaries, and the blood that fills them — nourishes your body and connects each part of the body to every other part. The cardiovascular system carries

- ✔ **Food** in the form of carbohydrates, protein, fat, vitamins, and minerals and brought in through the gastrointestinal tract to every organ in the body.

- ✔ **Oxygen,** brought in through the lungs and dissolved in the blood, to organs far from the lungs.

- ✔ **Waste,** a normal product of your body's metabolism that results from the many chemical reactions that are taking place in your body. For example, the cardiovascular system carries carbon dioxide to the lungs and the other waste products to the liver and kidneys.

Pressure must exist to push the blood through the cardiovascular system. Otherwise, on standing, your blood would pool in your legs and stay there due to gravity.

Just as your modern household water supply gets to you because pressure is pushing water through the pipes, the blood gets to your brain because pressure is allowing it to defy gravity and rise from the heart. The heart muscle, the source of this pressure, squeezes out the blood forcefully so the blood not only defies gravity but goes through the smallest passageways (the capillaries) that allow for exchanges, such as the release of oxygen and the uptake of carbon dioxide between the blood and the tissues through which it's passing.

When essential body organs, such as the kidneys, don't receive enough pressure to allow them to function properly, they signal the heart to pump harder. But what's good for the kidneys may not be good for the brain or the blood vessels themselves. That's when the consequences of high blood pressure occur (described in Chapter 3).

Comprehending the Numbers

When your doctor says, "Your blood pressure is 135 over 85," for example, what do the numbers really mean?

The first number is the *systolic blood pressure* (SBP) — the amount of pressure in your arteries as the heart pumps. *Systole* is the rhythmic contraction of your heart muscle when it's expelling blood from your left ventricle — the large chamber on the left side of your heart. The aortic valve sits between that chamber and your *aorta,* the large artery that takes blood away from the heart to the rest of the body. During systole, the aortic valve is open and blood flows freely to the rest of your body.

The second number is the *diastolic blood pressure* (DBP). After your heart empties the blood from the ventricle, the aortic valve shuts to prevent blood from returning into the heart from the rest of your body. Your heart muscle relaxes and the ventricle expands as blood fills it up from the left atrium, which has received it from the lungs. Within your arteries, the blood pressure rapidly falls until it reaches its lowest point. The diastolic blood pressure — the second number that's read on the gauge or the top of the mercury column reflects this lowest point of blood pressure. Before it falls further, the ventricle contracts again and the blood pressure starts to rise back up to the systolic level.

After you've established your SBP and DBP, determine whether your blood pressure is high and whether it should be treated. But first, how high is too high?

At birth, your blood pressure is around 90/60 mm Hg or even lower. As you grow older, it gradually rises until as an adult your blood pressure is generally between 120/80 mm Hg and 139/89 mm Hg. Higher than that and you're considered to have high blood pressure.

No fixed number serves as a guide for your diastolic or systolic blood pressure that tells you your blood pressure is high if it's above the number or low if it's below the number. Doctors established 140/90 mm Hg as the point at which action is taken, but the fact remains that a person with a blood pressure reading of 120/80 mm Hg is at lower risk of blood pressure complications than a person with a 130/85 mm Hg.

The National Heart, Lung, and Blood Institute, a division of the National Institutes of Health, established the Joint National Committee on Prevention, Detection, Evaluation, and Treatment of High Blood Pressure. The committee created a Classification of Blood Pressure for Adults that's shown in Table 1-1. Use the table to determine whether your blood pressure measurement is normal or abnormal. If your blood pressure falls in the high-normal or high blood pressure categories, discuss treatment with your doctor.

Note: When SBP and DBP fall into different categories, use the higher category. Also, Hg is the chemical notation for mercury.

Table 1-1 Classification of Blood Pressure for Adults*

Category	SBP (mm Hg)		DBP (mm Hg)
Optimal	<120	and	<80
Normal	<130	and	<85
High-normal	130–139	or	85–89
Stage 1 HBP	140–159	or	90–99
Stage 2 HBP	160–179	or	100–109
Stage 3 HBP	180+	or	110+

*As noted by the Joint National Committee on Prevention, Detection, Evaluation, and Treatment of High Blood Pressure.

Getting the Right Post-Diagnosis

If, by chance, you're unable to prevent yourself from developing high blood pressure, you want to make sure that your doctor evaluates your blood pressure properly. Assuming this is a first visit to the doctor for established high blood pressure, the doctor must make a number of assessments that can be categorized as history, physical examination, and lab testing.

Assessing your history

Your history describes your past association with high blood pressure. It's similar to a history taken for any other condition with a few variations specific to high blood pressure. The important points in the history are

- Duration of high blood pressure (when it was first discovered)

- Course of the blood pressure (whether it has always been high since it was discovered)

- Treatment with drugs, diet, exercise, or other means

- Use of agents that could worsen blood pressure, such as steroids, birth control pills, and nonsteroidal anti-inflammatory agents

- Any family history of high blood pressure

- Symptoms that may suggest secondary high blood pressure

- Symptoms of the consequences of high blood pressure

- Presence of other risk factors, such as smoking, diabetes, and high cholesterol

- Social factors, such as family structure, work, and education

✔ Dietary history

✔ Sexual function (to evaluate before using drugs that affect it)

✔ Possibility of sleep apnea (a condition in which an individual gasps for breath and snores during sleep following several stops in breathing)

Evaluating your physical exam

After the doctor notes the history, she should do a physical examination. This is also mostly a routine evaluation with some special studies because of the high blood pressure. The main parts of the exam are

✔ Abdominal exam to look for tumors or abnormal sounds suggesting restricted blood flow

✔ Blood pressure reading as described earlier in this chapter

✔ Body fat distribution

✔ Examination of the neck for thyroid or blood vessel abnormalities

✔ Examination of the pulses in the arteries

✔ Heart exam

✔ Internal eye exam

✔ Lung exam

✔ Neurological exam

Sending samples to the lab

Your history and physical exam can give the doctor an excellent idea of the severity of the problem and the possibility that secondary high blood pressure is present. Then lab tests are used to get a general picture of your overall health and to look for specific abnormalities that the history and physical pointed to. The key lab tests done on everyone with high blood pressure are

- ✔ Complete blood count
- ✔ Serum chemistry profile that looks at the sodium, potassium, liver function, and the kidney function.
- ✔ Lipid profile that evaluates cholesterol and triglycerides
- ✔ Microalbumin test to look for early kidney disease

If definite damage associated with high blood pressure is suspected, the doctor should do other studies. For example:

- ✔ **Brain abnormalities:** The doctor might do a study called a Doppler flow study to check for blockage of blood vessels in the neck.
- ✔ **Heart disease:** Do an electrocardiogram and chest X-ray.
- ✔ **Kidney problems:** Check for increased uric acid using a blood test.

Examining the Risk Factors for High Blood Pressure

A tremendous effort has been made to understand the cause of high blood pressure and what populations are at risk of developing the disease. Numerous unalterable factors affect blood pressure (such as age, sex, ethnic background, and family history), and to some extent, how these factors can contribute to high blood pressure is understood. But which of these factors is the major factor is unknown.

Certain changeable factors (such as diet, exercise routine, and stress) can also place you at risk of developing high blood pressure. Ask yourself the following questions:

- ✔ Am I less active than I could be in my day-to-day routine?
- ✔ Am I overweight?
- ✔ Do I eat many salty foods?
- ✔ Do I have a stressful lifestyle?
- ✔ Do I smoke? Drink?

If you answered "Yes" to any one of these questions, then you're at risk of developing high blood pressure. The more questions that you answer in the affirmative, the greater your odds are for developing high blood pressure. If you decrease the stress in your life and keep a rein on these changeable factors, you can decrease the possibility of developing high blood pressure.

Ninety-five percent of high blood pressure is categorized as *essential high blood pressure* (but "primary high blood pressure" would be a better term) because what's causing the elevated pressure is unknown. In all other cases, a specific disease is identifiable that, when treated, usually normalizes the blood pressure. This is *secondary high blood pressure*. I discuss some causes of secondary high blood pressure (such as kidney disease and adrenal gland tumors) in Chapter 2.

Reviewing the Consequences of High Blood Pressure

High blood pressure can wreak havoc on your heart, kidneys, and brain, if untreated. Heart attacks and/or heart failure may be the major consequence for your heart. Kidney failure may affect your kidneys. A brain attack (stroke) may destroy important brain tissue and the movements it controls in the body. I discuss these consequences in Chapter 3.

Deaths due to these conditions do occur, but the greater majority of those who have serious conditions resulting from high blood pressure suffer debilitating illness. Of those who survive a massive heart attack, kidney failure, or brain attack, many require the care of others for the rest of their lives.

Most of this sickness and death due to high blood pressure is preventable. Chapters 4 through 6 give you the tools you need to accomplish this. It may be costly in terms of your time and your resources, but the savings in freedom from illness and a longer life is worth it

Treating High Blood Pressure

Treating high blood pressure involves making use of all the tools discussed in this book. Switching from a diet that promotes high blood pressure to a diet that lowers blood pressure — from a diet that's high in salt and fats to a diet that emphasizes grains, fruits, and vegetables, changes your lifestyle for the better.

Then add regular exercise to this. A program of daily aerobic exercise (see Chapter 6) is not excessive, but it should be done at least four times a week.

Cardiac output and peripheral resistance

An increase in blood volume creates an increase in cardiac output. An increase in blood volume results from salt intake, for example, which causes water retention. More blood volume may be present in the central part of the body and less in the peripheral part. The body doesn't permit the cardiac output to remain elevated. It lowers the cardiac output by increasing the peripheral resistance. The blood vessels constrict so that too much blood doesn't flow through the tissues. This rise in peripheral resistance leads to increased blood pressure.

A minor alteration in body chemistry may be enough to cause persistent high blood pressure. For example, a slight increase in angiotensin II, a hormone produced when the kidney detects a low blood pressure, may cause thickening and narrowing of the blood vessels that then leads to sustained high blood pressure. Other hormones, called *growth factors,* can lead to narrow arteries and increased peripheral resistance as well.

On the other hand, a chemical called *nitric oxide,* made in the endothelial cells that line the inside of the blood vessels, is the most potent cause of widening in blood vessels. If anything blocks the production of nitric oxide, the blood pressure rises. It's known that nitric oxide is reduced in essential high blood pressure, and this may be a further cause of the increased peripheral resistance.

Next, eliminate the poisons, such as tobacco, excessive alcohol, and some caffeine (see Chapter 5). At this point, you may have done enough to lower your pressure to normal. If not, you have the option of adding one or more drugs (see Chapter 7). Drugs shouldn't be a substitute for improvements in your lifestyle, but *in addition* to lifestyle changes.

Staying Informed

Myths about high blood pressure and its treatment are numerous. I take up only ten in Chapter 8, but I tried to find the myths that are most often believed and are most detrimental to your health. If you know of a myth that you think is damaging to many people with high blood pressure, by all means e-mail me at `highbloodpressure@drrubin.com` and let me know.

Chapter 2

Understanding Secondary High Blood Pressure

* *

In This Chapter

▶ Discovering secondary high blood pressure early on

▶ Dealing with renal vascular high blood pressure

▶ Finding a tumor that induces secondary high blood pressure

▶ Regulating an overabundance of cortisol

▶ Coping with causes that you're born with and more

* *

*S*econdary high blood pressure means that a specific disease causes the high blood pressure — the high blood pressure is one of several signs and symptoms associated with the disease. If you're cured of the disease that's causing the secondary high blood pressure, then the high blood pressure is lowered. Treatment of the disease often eliminates the high blood pressure.

Although secondary high blood pressure makes up only 5 percent of the total number of high blood pressure cases, its causes are important. A careful history, physical exam, and lab evaluation can help a physician discover the disease that's causing your blood pressure to rise. This chapter introduces you to some of the most common causes of secondary high blood pressure.

The upside of secondary high blood pressure is that after the disease that's causing it is identified and treated, you're like new most of the time. The high blood pressure and the other signs and symptoms of the disease disappear. Your whole life will improve.

Nipping Secondary High Blood Pressure in the Bud

Several clues that should prompt an investigation for secondary high blood pressure include

- ✔ Damage to the eyes, kidneys, or heart
- ✔ Family history of kidney disease
- ✔ Flushing spells when your skin turns red and hot
- ✔ Increased body pigmentation and pigmented stretch marks
- ✔ Intolerance to heat
- ✔ Loud humming sound in the abdomen (called a *bruit*)
- ✔ Low potassium level in the blood
- ✔ Poor response to usually effective treatment for high blood pressure
- ✔ Rapid pulse

✔ The onset of high blood pressure before age 20 or past age 50

✔ Unusually high level of high blood pressure (above 180/120 mm Hg)

If you notice any of the clues in the preceding list, talk to your doctor. By finding and treating secondary high blood pressure early, you're more certain to have a return to normal blood pressure before permanent changes occur. Some changes, such as kidney damage, can affect your high blood pressure permanently even if the disease or disorder that's causing the secondary high blood pressure is eliminated.

Secondary High Blood Pressure and Your Kidneys

At some point or other, the kidneys get involved when high blood pressure is present. Damage to the kidneys may precede the high blood pressure. Then the high blood pressure is secondary. If the high blood pressure precedes the kidney damage, the high blood pressure is primary or *essential.* Two main conditions of the kidney, damaged kidney tissue and blocked kidney arteries, can lead to high blood pressure.

Discovering damaged kidney tissue

Damaged kidney tissue is the most common reason for secondary high blood pressure, accounting for about 50 percent of the cases.

Renal (kidney) *parenchymal* (tissue) *hypertension* (high blood pressure) results from a kidney-damaging illness such as diabetes, use of certain medications, an inflammation of the kidney, or a hereditary disease that results in *cysts* (sacs filled with fluid). The damaged kidneys don't function normally and can't eliminate sodium at a normal rate, resulting in salt and water retention that leads to high blood pressure.

Loss of kidney tissue that leads to high blood pressure can be *chronic* (slow to develop) or *acute* (sudden). Some of the diseases and conditions that cause chronic kidney damage are

- Chronic obstruction of the *ureter* (the tube that takes urine from the kidney to the bladder)
- Cysts that displace normal kidney tissue
- Damage to the *glomerulus* (the filtering part of the kidney)
- Diabetes mellitus (diabetic kidney disease)

Controlling the secondary high blood pressure present in all the conditions in the preceding list is important because continued high blood pressure acting on the kidneys can damage the kidneys further and lead to even higher blood pressure. It's a vicious cycle.

High blood pressure also accompanies acute kidney diseases, such as blockage in the arteries to both kidneys, trauma to the kidneys, or after certain X-ray or surgical procedures. For example, certain chemicals used to observe the kidneys during an X-ray may suddenly damage the kidneys, especially in people with diabetes. Surgery that accidentally damages the arteries to the kidneys also leads to a sudden rise in blood pressure. Most of them resolve over time if the person is given the necessary medical support during the acute illness.

The details of diabetic kidney disease

Diabetes mellitus, a particularly damaging disease that may affect the kidneys, is the most common cause of kidney damage and kidney failure. It usually takes 15 or more years of poorly controlled diabetes to reach the point of affecting the kidneys. Most people who have diabetes mellitus also have high blood pressure and *diabetic retinopathy,* the characteristic eye disease seen in diabetes. Certain drugs called *ACE inhibitors* (see Chapter 7) are particularly helpful in slowing the progression of diabetic kidney disease and may even reverse it.

In diabetic kidney disease, the most important treatments consist of controlling blood glucose (sugar), blood pressure, and blood cholesterol. Diabetics should restrict their salt intake as well as their protein, which seems to make the kidney disease worse.

Dealing with blocked kidney arteries

Diseases that cause *renal* (kidney) *vascular* (blood vessel) *hypertension* (high blood pressure), a block to one or both kidney arteries, bring on high blood pressure through the production of an enzyme called *renin.* The kidney that isn't receiving enough blood flow because of the obstruction secretes renin. The renin, in turn, raises the blood pressure through its action on a hormone called *angiotensin I* to produce *angiotensin II,* a hormone that causes the contraction of blood vessels. Angiotensin II also stimulates the production of *aldosterone,* a hormone that causes salt and water retention. Because of the obstruction, the increased blood pressure is still unable to cause more blood flow in the obstructed kidney, and the high blood pressure continues.

Many diseases can cause obstruction of one or both of the kidney arteries. These diseases occur in about 6 out of 100,000 people. Among them are

- ✔ **Atherosclerosis:** The process by which cholesterol is laid down in the arteries and eventually leads to narrowing of the arteries. This is usually seen in men over the age of 45 and accounts for two-thirds of cases.

- ✔ **Fibromuscular disease:** The kidney artery and the body's arteries in general become thickened and narrowed, especially in young women under the age of 45 and in children who have the disease.

- ✔ **Aneurysms:** The kidney artery or the heart's aorta (the artery leading to the kidney's artery) can have a defect and balloon out, thus causing blockage. Then blood enters the wall of the artery and the normal passage through which blood flows narrows. The great danger of aneurysms is bursting.

- ✔ **Emboli-clots:** Blood clots that block the artery.

Hormone-Secreting Tumors That Elevate Blood Pressure

Certain tumors produce hormones (chemical messengers that trigger reactions) that elevate blood pressure to an abnormal extent. These tumors form in organs that make these hormones normally in small amounts. These tumors usually originate in an *adrenal gland,* but these tumors can also arise in nerve tissues. (You have two adrenal glands — one adrenal gland sits on top of each of your kidneys.) The adrenal glands secrete the following hormones:

- ✔ **Epinephrine:** Maintains blood pressure and blood glucose

> ✔ **Aldosterone:** Controls salt and water levels in the bloodstream

> ✔ **Cortisol:** Maintains blood glucose (sugar) and also plays a role in maintaining blood pressure

Finding an epinephrine-producing tumor

Epinephrine (adrenaline), a normal product of the adrenal gland, raises blood pressure, heart rate, and blood glucose during stressful times and causes sweating. Sometimes a *pheochromocytoma* (a tumor that releases large quantities of epinephrine) can arise in an adrenal gland or along many nerves.

Forms of pheochromocytoma run in families as solitary pheochromocytoma or along with other tumors. When several different tumors are present the condition is *multiple endocrine neoplasia* and comes in several types, each of which involves the addition of other tumors in other glands to the pheochromocytoma. Tumors of the thyroid gland and the parathyroid gland should be looked for whenever a pheochromocytoma is discovered.

Detecting a tumor that produces aldosterone

The *adrenal cortex* (the outer covering of the adrenal gland) secretes *aldosterone,* an important hormone that's responsible for retaining salt and eliminating potassium from the body. A malfunction of the adrenal gland called *primary hyperaldosteronism* (usually due to an aldosterone-producing tumor in one of the adrenal glands) may produce an overabundance of aldosterone — more than the human body can handle safely.

A large amount of aldosterone causes significant sodium retention and potassium loss to the point that the blood potassium is low. It also causes high blood pressure.

The incidence of aldosterone-producing tumors is 2 out of 100,000 people. However, some high blood pressure specialists believe that the prevalence of primary hyperaldosteronism is much greater than generally accepted and suggest that

- ✔ As many as one in ten people with high blood pressure have primary hyperaldosteronism although not necessarily due to a tumor.

- ✔ Primary hyperaldosteronism should be considered in every case of high blood pressure even when the potassium is normal.

- ✔ Testing for the aldosterone level and the renin level in the bloodstream and getting the ratio of aldosterone to renin is recommended.

Aldosterone-producing tumors are usually found in people between the ages of 30 and 50, and women are affected more often than men.

Because the blood pressure can be so high, those who suffer from an aldosterone-producing tumor may develop a brain attack, damage to the kidneys, or an enlarged heart before the disease is treated. The low potassium level in the bloodstream can lead to a reduced secretion of insulin and diabetes as well as muscle weakness.

Investigating Cushing's Syndrome

As if the previous two tumors weren't enough trouble from the adrenal gland, the adrenal gland can be the site of still another source of secondary high blood pressure, namely *Cushing's syndrome*. This syndrome results whenever the adrenal glands make too much cortisol (the main hormone made by the adrenal glands), which can occur in three different ways:

- ✔ The pituitary hormone that regulates the adrenal gland stimulates the adrenals.

- ✔ A tumor grows within one adrenal gland.

- ✔ Rarely, an adrenal-stimulating hormone coming from some other tumor in the body stimulates the adrenals.

The overabundance of cortisol usually (about 80 percent of the time) results from an excessive production of *adrenocorticotrophin* (ACTH) — the hormone that regulates the adrenal glands — coming from the pituitary gland in the brain. The ACTH stimulates both adrenals to make too much cortisol.

The remaining 20 percent of the time, one adrenal gland has a tumor that makes too much cortisol. Normally, the adrenal gland is under the control of ACTH from the brain. If a tumor forms in the part of the brain that makes ACTH, the pituitary gland, it can cause the adrenals to make too much cortisol as well as other steroids that have plenty of salt-retaining activity, and the blood pressure rises. When the adrenal tumor makes too much cortisol independently of ACTH, ACTH is suppressed instead of elevated.

Cushing's syndrome is associated with high blood pressure that's difficult to treat. The pressure may be up to 200/120 mm Hg. The death rate from untreated Cushing's syndrome is high. It occurs three times as often in women as men, usually in the third or fourth decade of an individual's life.

Realizing a Genetic Disease Is Causing High Blood Pressure

Congenital adrenal hyperplasia, an inherited disease, is the genetic lack of one or more enzymes that are needed to change steroids from one form to another and eventually to cortisol in the adrenal glands. This leads to an overproduction of other hormones that have properties similar to aldosterone. When the pituitary gland does not detect sufficient cortisol, it sends out more ACTH to stimulate the adrenals, which then enlarge. The two most common forms of congenital adrenal hyperplasia are as follows:

✔ In one form of congenital adrenal hyperplasia, the excessive steroids are both aldosterone-like, producing high blood pressure and low potassium, and masculinizing, causing masculine changes in baby girls, so that their genital organs are something between male and female. A milder form can present itself in such a way that the onset of puberty in boys is early. The symptomatic increase of male hormone activity, such as increased hair and menstrual irregularity, can also occur in young girls.

✔ In a second form of congenital adrenal hyperplasia, the excessive steroids are again aldosterone-like, causing high blood pressure and low potassium, but no sex hormones are made at all. When the female is supposed to begin menstruation, it doesn't take place, so the disease is first detected at puberty. Lack of male hormone in boys leads to abnormal development of the male sexual organs, which is found earlier than in the case of the girls.

Although these conditions are rare, they're easily treated if diagnosed early. The patients are simply given cortisol, which shuts off the excessive ACTH and the production of the abnormal steroids. In the second form of congenital adrenal hyperplasia, sex hormones must be given to replace the absent hormones. Because these diseases are hereditary, they're found in certain groups more often than others. This alerts doctors to look for the condition whenever a new birth occurs in one of these groups.

Other Causes of Secondary High Blood Pressure

Several other treatable diseases can be associated with high blood pressure. These diseases need to be considered because most of them are reversible, and the high blood pressure responds to the correction of the disease unless it's been present for some time.

✔ *Coarctation of the aorta* is a narrowing of the large artery that leaves the heart. Depending on how severe the narrowing is, the narrowing is usually present at birth though not diagnosed until the teenage years. The narrowing is usually in an area soon after the beginning of the aorta but below where the artery branches off to supply blood to the arms. The result is that the blood pressure in the arms is high and the blood pressure in the legs is lower.

The kidneys are also exposed to the lower blood pressure and respond by putting out more of the enzyme renin, leading to even higher blood pressure above the narrowing but not below it.

✔ Both *hyperthyroidism* (too much thyroid hormone) and *hypothyroidism* (too little thyroid hormone) can be associated with high blood pressure. These conditions may be easy to diagnose if the symptoms are significant, but hypothyroidism is often subtle.

✔ *Acromegaly* results from a slow-growing tumor of the pituitary gland that makes too much growth hormone. Among other things, the growth hormone causes sodium retention and high blood pressure.

✔ *Sleep apnea* is a condition in which an individual gasps for breath and snores during sleep following several stops in breathing. It's significant when it happens five or more times in an hour. Because the lack of breathing occurs many times, the person has a reduction in blood oxygen and an increase in carbon dioxide in the blood. The decrease in oxygen causes constriction of the blood vessels with resultant high blood pressure. These people have also been found to have increased heart disease.

✔ Brain tumors increase pressure within the brain and the blood pressure throughout the body.

✔ Severe burns are associated with high blood pressure in about 25 percent of burn cases. The high stress associated with the burn causes the high blood pressure. A bad burn also triggers the release of hormones that cause blood vessel constriction.

Chapter 3

Considering the Medical Consequences

. . . .

In This Chapter

▶ Following your blood through the heart

▶ Looking at various diseases that affect the heart

▶ Figuring out when your heart is failing and how

▶ Looking into damage to the kidneys

▶ Understanding stroke, or brain attack

. . . .

*T*hree major organs of the body suffer when high blood pressure isn't controlled: the heart, the kidneys, and the brain. In this chapter, I explain exactly how high blood pressure affects each of these organs and how the sooner any damage is diagnosed, the better the chances are of reversing the damage. I also address ways to deal with organ damage that may have already resulted from high blood pressure.

Uncontrolled high blood pressure tends to damage the heart, kidneys, and brain together and within the same time frame.

It's been said that gambling is a great way of getting nothing for something, and you can gamble away your life if you don't control your blood pressure — this is guaranteed.

Introducing the Mighty Pump

What a piece of work is the heart! An organ that's mostly muscle, your heart is about the size of your clenched fist and weighs about 10½ ounces. This little muscle is responsible for supplying blood and oxygen to all parts of your body, which is usually 15 or more times as heavy as the heart itself.

Your heart is in your chest cavity behind your breastbone and between your lungs. The heart is divided into four chambers, the left and right atria and the left and right ventricles. The right atrium receives blood through the veins called *vena cava* and pushes it into the right ventricle. The right ventricle squeezes down and sends the blood into the pulmonary arteries to the lungs where the blood picks up oxygen. Pulmonary veins carry the blood back to the left atrium, which sends it down to the left ventricle. The left ventricle squeezes the blood into a major artery, the aorta, which sends it to every cell and organ. Valves that close, blocking backward flow, prevent the blood from going backwards from the left side of the heart to the lungs, from the right side of the heart to the veins, and from the ventricles to the atria.

This amazing pump pushes 1½ gallons of blood forward every minute. Every hour, it sends 90 gallons around the body, enough to fill the gas tanks in most cars six times, assuming a 15-gallon gas tank. In a day that you spend mostly resting, your heart pumps 2,160 gallons of blood. If you're working or playing energetically, the number gets much higher.

The combination of the heart, the blood vessels that carry the blood, and the blood itself is the *cardiovascular system*.

When the blood pressure rises, the heart must work harder to push the blood through. It was not meant to have to struggle so hard and eventually it may fail, a condition where the heart muscles are just too tired and weak to work properly.

Blocking Blood Flow to the Heart Muscle

Just like any other organ of the body, your heart muscle must receive oxygen, *glucose* (blood sugar), and other nutrients in order to work. These nutrients are the food of the heart muscles. When the bloodstream that carries these nutrients is partially obstructed (called *arteriosclerosis*) so that the heart muscle is partially starving, the heart muscle can cause pain. If the obstruction remains about the same, the pain is stable. A complete obstruction causes a heart attack, which is the death of heart muscle tissue.

Examining arteriosclerosis

Arteriosclerosis is hardening of the arteries — the process that leads to obstruction of arteries throughout the body as a result of deposition of cholesterol and formation of a plaque, a narrowing of an artery that blocks the flow of blood. (See the "Formation of a plaque" sidebar in this chapter.) When the blood flow is blocked, the heart has to pump harder, leading to thickening of the heart muscles called *hypertrophy*.

High blood pressure can increase the development of fatty deposits in the walls of the arteries leading to

- ✔ **Atherosclerosis:** A form of arteriosclerosis in the medium- to large-size arteries
- ✔ **Arteriolosclerosis:** Arteriosclerosis in the small arteries
- ✔ **Coronary atherosclerosis:** Involves the arteries to the muscle of the heart

As the coronary arteries (the ones that feed the heart muscle) become more and more blocked, the heart muscle may be hungry for nutrients or even die, a condition called *coronary artery disease* (also known as *coronary heart disease* and *atherosclerotic heart disease*).

According to the National Institutes of Health, one of every six deaths (425,425 total) in the United States each year is the result of atherosclerosis of the arteries to the heart, resulting in a lethal heart attack. In addition to these deaths, another 830,000 people have heart attacks but don't die for a total of about 1.255 million. About 17½ million people in the United States have chest pain associated with coronary atherosclerosis, a heart attack, or some other form of coronary atherosclerosis. Due to the greater prevalence of high blood pressure among the African American population, this group has a higher rate of coronary heart disease than any other ethnic group.

Formation of a plaque

When high blood pressure, smoking, diabetes and/or increased levels of cholesterol, especially low-density lipoprotein (LDL) cholesterol, damage the inner lining of the arteries, a plaque begins to form.

After damage has occurred, fat begins to accumulate within a part of the artery wall called the *intima*. In the intima, fat is protected from the chemicals in the blood that prevent changes in the fat, and it begins to change to a more damaging form.

White blood cells, especially monocytes and lymphocytes that enter the intima from the blood, are transformed into other cells called *macrophages,* and the macrophages begin gobbling up the changed fat to turn the cells into *foam cells.* Calcium is also deposited in the walls where the plaque is forming and is responsible for the calcification seen in arteries when X-rays are taken.

This accumulation of foam cells and calcium is now called plaque. It grows and begins to stick out into the *lumen* (the hollow part inside) of the artery. After 80 percent of the lumen is blocked, blood flow to the heart muscle is reduced.

The irregular surface of a plaque can be the site of accumulation of blood platelets and the formation of a clot. The clot can go on and reduce the opening of the lumen even more at that position, or it can break off and lodge in a smaller artery, completely closing off blood flow beyond it.

Atherosclerotic heart disease (coronary artery disease) is found in the arteries of people who die as young as age twenty, or even younger of other causes, and is extensive in older people who die of other causes. However, it's not found in everyone. Those who don't have risk factors, such as uncontrolled high blood pressure, cigarette smoking, diabetes, a sedentary lifestyle, and high cholesterol levels, rarely have problems with coronary artery disease. A family history of coronary artery disease is another risk factor and one that you can do nothing about, but its effect is minimized when the other risk factors are avoided or controlled.

Coronary artery disease may cause sudden death as the first sign of the presence of the disease in as many as 25 percent of the patients. Another 20 percent die before they reach the hospital as a result of a fatal irregularity in their heartbeat. The rest may undergo a procedure to try to open the blocked artery or arteries.

Managing stable heart pain

Stable heart pain, pain that doesn't get worse over time, due to coronary atherosclerosis, is *angina pectoris* (Latin for "pain in the chest"). Angina pectoris (commonly known as *angina*) affects 10.2 million people in the United States. Not only is angina pectoris the result of blockage of an artery, but it can also be brought on if the coronary artery squeezes down, for example, after a meal when blood is diverted to the intestine, thus causing a decrease in blood supply to the heart.

Some diseases like hyperthyroidism (stemming from an overactive thyroid gland), which increases the demands on the body's metabolism, can cause angina even in the absence of coronary atherosclerosis. The right coronary artery supplies blood to the right side of the heart. The left main coronary artery supplies the left side of the heart. It, in turn, divides into the left anterior descending artery that supplies the front of the left side and the left circumflex artery that curves around to the back. Both the left and right coronary arteries begin as the left ventricle continues into the aorta, the major artery carrying blood away from the heart to the rest of the body.

Treating an acute heart attack

A heart attack, also known as a *myocardial infarction* (MI), where heart muscle tissue dies because it lacks a supply of blood, can cause immediate death in 25 percent of the people who have one, and another 20 percent never reach the hospital alive. For those who do make it to the hospital, however, excellent treatment is available.

The symptoms that suggest that an individual is having a heart attack include the following:

- ✔ Development of severe pain in the front of the chest that lasts for more than 30 minutes with radiation down the left arm

- ✔ Unexplained shock, a severe fall in blood pressure, sometimes accompanied by vomiting and even unconsciousness

- ✔ A feeling of impending doom with sweating and a rapid heart beat

Call 911 for an ambulance ride to the nearest hospital, and call your doctor for follow-up.

The doctor will question you to find out if there has been a recent change in your pattern of chest pain. He'll ask whether you're experiencing sweating, dizziness, nausea, and weakness.

Your blood pressure may be low. You may appear pale. Your heart rhythm may be irregular. On examination, your chest may have *rales,* the sound of fluid in the lungs as a result of some *heart failure* (when your heart isn't able to pump enough blood to maintain an adequate flow to and from the body tissues). Your heart may reveal soft sounds that mean the muscle isn't functioning properly.

The doctor does lab studies, which may show the following:

- Elevations of heart enzymes, chemicals usually found only in the heart that leak into the blood when the heart muscle is damaged

- Electrocardiographic changes that suggest a heart attack

- Changes in the movement of the heart wall, so that when the wall should be moving in to squeeze out blood, it doesn't move or flops outward

One of the biggest advances in the treatment of heart attacks is the availability of *thrombolytic therapy,* drugs that dissolve the clot that's obstructing the coronary artery and that allow blood to flow back into the obstructed area. This decreases the size of the damage and often saves the patient. A possible side effect of thrombolytic therapy is the danger of bleeding in undesired areas such as the brain, especially if the blood pressure isn't controlled.

Several different agents are used for thrombolytic therapy. The choice depends on your doctor's experience with each of them. The success of this treatment depends on how quickly the patient gets to the doctor after the onset of the heart attack, and the earlier, the better. The reopening may be as much as 80 percent. This reopening accompanies an end to the pain and an improved EKG reading.

The blood vessel closes again in 10 percent of cases, and then surgery must be done to permanently reopen the artery. Sometimes the thrombolytic therapy isn't done in favor of immediate surgery, especially in the severely sick patient with a heart attack and shock.

After the initial treatment is given, the heart attack patient is observed in the coronary care unit for a couple of days. Then the patient gradually returns to normal activity. Studies have shown that several drugs can significantly reduce the chance of a future heart attack when they're prescribed early. Aspirin is administered to prevent more clots. Beta blockers have been shown to extend the life of the patient after a heart attack. If pain occurs, nitroglycerine remains the treatment of choice.

Developing Heart Failure

When high blood pressure is present, your heart is forced to pump against more resistance. It needs to sustain its output, so it must thicken to do so. Just like the muscles of a weight lifter, the heart muscle gets bigger and thicker. But heart muscle can only thicken so far. After a while, the heart enlarges to the point that it can no longer pump effectively and heart failure begins.

Comparing the statistics for the prevalence of heart failure today with 20 years ago, clearly, more heart failure is occurring today. Exactly why this is so isn't clear, but uncontrolled high blood pressure is certainly one contributing factor.

If you suffer from heart failure, you may experience angina pectoris (pain most often felt in the front of the chest) or it can be felt in the jaw, the left arm, or the shoulder. (Angina is described earlier in this

chapter in the "Managing stable heart pain" section.)
This comes from the high oxygen requirement of the
thick heart muscle plus the decreased blood supply
coming through the arteries that supply the heart.
At first, angina pain begins during activity. As the
condition worsens, it occurs when you're at rest.

Your doctor can tell that your heart is developing
problems because your heart sounds (that he can
hear in his stethoscope) change. When the doctor
puts his hand on the front of your chest, he feels a
thumping at the place where your heart beats against
the chest wall. As your heart fails, that thumping is
felt farther away from the center of your chest,
indicating that your heart is getting larger.

Noticing the telltale signs

The most common symptom of heart failure is difficulty
breathing, known as *dyspnea*. At first, breathing is
only difficult during exercise. As the heart failure
increases, however, the individual has difficulty
breathing when she's resting, too. People without
heart failure may get short of breath with exercise,
too, but only after exercising at least for a few minutes
or so. People whose hearts are failing have difficulty
breathing at the onset of exercising.

The reason that this symptom develops is that the
blood vessels of the failing heart become congested
with blood — sometimes even leaking into the lung
tissue. The lungs, ordinarily light and filled with air,
become much heavier. The diaphragm and the other
muscles of respiration have a much harder time
pushing air out and pulling it in. They become
fatigued, and this is felt as shortness of breath.

As the lungs fill with fluid, the patient is unable to lie down flat without raising his head. When flat, more blood pools in the lungs making breathing even more difficult. The patient may need to sleep on several pillows and should his head fall off the pillows, he may have a coughing spell. This symptom is *orthopnea,* and improves when the patient sits up or raises his head.

Ejection fraction — What's your function?

Assessing the *ejection fraction* is one of the best ways to measure your heart function. The *ejection fraction* is the ratio of the amount of blood that's pushed out of the heart with each beat, called the *stroke volume,* divided by the amount of blood within the large chamber of the heart (the left ventricle) when it's completely full, the *end diastolic volume.* If the ejection fraction is low, it means that a significant fraction of the blood in the left ventricle is left inside the heart with each beat, suggesting an inefficient (failing) heart. These volumes can be determined by an ultrasound study that uses the different echo properties of blood and heart tissue to produce a picture of the heart at rest (end diastolic volume) or when pumping (end systolic volume). The amount of blood at rest minus the amount after pumping, divided by the amount at rest, gives the ejection fraction. Alternately, an X-ray study can provide the same information.

Measurements while the patient is exercising may be even more helpful because this is the time when the heart is being maximally stressed. While nonstressed values may be normal, the patient may show evidence of significant heart failure when the heart is stressed.

Sometimes a severe coughing spell and shortness of breath that can't be relieved just by sitting up or raising the head can awaken the patient. This can be a terrifying experience because the patient can't catch his breath. This is *paroxysmal nocturnal dyspnea*. It's associated with an abundance of fluid in the lung tissue where it doesn't belong.

 Symptoms as severe as those felt in the condition of paroxysmal nocturnal dyspnea require a call to 911 and emergency room treatment.

Other signs and symptoms of heart failure that are less specific include:

✓ Fatigue and weakness

✓ Confused mental state due to poor blood flow to the brain

 Severe shortness of breath, mental confusion, severe fatigue, or the new onset of chest pain require a visit to your doctor.

Treating heart failure

After heart failure is diagnosed, it's up to your doctor to give you the information and the drugs that you need to manage the condition. This is a complicated process and won't be discussed in detail here. (See *Heart Disease For Dummies* by James M. Rippe, MD [Wiley] for more information on this treatment.) However, like all illness, successful treatment depends on your willingness to follow the doctor's recommendations. Some of your doctor's instructions and treatments may include the following:

✓ Significant reduction in salt intake, not just to lower blood pressure but even more to prevent water retention associated with increased salt

> ✔ Use of certain medications including ACE
> inhibitors to lower blood pressure and reduce
> salt and water retention, diuretics to eliminate
> salt and water through the kidneys, vasodilators
> to open the arteries, or digitalis to increase the
> heart muscle's ability to contract
>
> ✔ Restriction of activity to give the heart a rest
>
> ✔ Weight loss to reduce the work of the heart
>
> ✔ Reduction of fluid intake

Digging into Kidney Damage

Your kidneys are truly amazing. Kidneys filter the
blood, which acts much like a cargo carrier, dropping
off nutrients and picking up waste from all the cells
everywhere in your body. The blood carries waste
from the cells to your body's waste-disposal head-
quarters — the kidneys. Separating out the recyclable
material from the trash that needs to pass on to the
bladder and out the urethra, the kidneys filter out
what can be reused from what needs to be passed off
in the form of urine.

Your kidneys filter an enormous amount of blood
every minute, namely one and one-half quarts. They
don't allow blood cells (such as your red blood cells
and white blood cells) and large chemical compounds
to pass through the filter, but everything else, including
the toxins (waste products of normal metabolism)
is filtered. The kidneys reabsorb the recyclable
materials — 99 percent of the desired water, sodium,
and other key body elements — back into the body. A
little water carries the toxins to the bladder as urine;
then the urine passes out of the body through the
urethra.

How untreated high blood pressure affects the kidneys

Before medications for high blood pressure control were available, a great number of subjects (people with uncontrolled high blood pressure) were studied and followed. After 15 to 25 years of no control, abnormally high levels of protein (an indication of kidney damage) were found in the urine of about 40 percent of the subjects. After this was discovered, these subjects died in about 5 years. Those subjects that had an elevation in blood urea nitrogen (evidence of kidney function loss because the kidney ordinarily eliminates this) lived about another year. A typical study can be found in the *Journal of Chronic Diseases* (January 1955) where 500 patients were followed for an average of 20 years.

After an individual is diagnosed with end-stage renal disease, life expectancy is now prolonged due in part to dialysis and kidney transplantation. Currently, about 10 percent of deaths associated with high blood pressure are due to kidney failure.

The process requires pressure to force the liquid part of the blood through, so the kidney has a built-in mechanism that maintains the necessary level of blood pressure should it decline. Too much pressure for too much time causes damage. If the damage proceeds, the result is end-stage renal disease. If a patient has end-stage renal disease, his kidneys can't filter the blood and eliminate toxins without the help of dialysis or transplantation.

Managing malignant high blood pressure

Malignant high blood pressure (often found in smokers and in young African American males) affects about 1 percent of people with high blood pressure. It refers to severely high blood pressure with a diastolic reading often greater than 150 mm Hg along with evidence of severe complications including:

✔ Severe eye damage, and even blindness

✔ Progressive damage to the brain that may manifest itself as headaches to start with. Next, the individual with malignant high blood pressure may become confused and finally lapse into a coma.

✔ Rapid development of partial or total loss of kidney function

✔ Nausea and vomiting

Dramatically elevated blood pressure isn't enough to make a malignant high blood pressure diagnosis. People with the same high blood pressure reading may not have the condition. The symptoms in the preceding list are necessary to make the diagnosis.

The exact cause of malignant high blood pressure is unclear. Malignant high blood pressure may be the direct result of poor blood pressure control. The blood pressure is allowed to rise to this dangerous level. Additional explanations include the production of chemicals by damaged kidneys. These chemicals further damage the kidney and cause contraction of blood vessels, thus raising the blood pressure. Other chemicals that usually widen blood vessels may be suppressed.

Causes of secondary high blood pressure (see Chapter 2), especially *renal artery stenosis,* also trigger malignant high blood pressure in as many as one third of cases.

In the days before 1950 or so, when treatment for high blood pressure wasn't available, the majority of these patients were dead within six months. Now that effective treatment is available, the response to treatment depends on how much irreversible kidney damage has taken place. The treatment consists of lowering the blood pressure. If the kidney damage is minimal, then more than 90 percent of patients are alive after five years. Even among those with kidney damage, the survival is about 65 percent after five years. If these patients don't have a fatal heart attack, the eventual cause of death in these patients is end-stage renal disease, particularly if their kidneys show signs of damage.

Coping with end-stage renal disease

End-stage renal disease (ESRD), also known as *chronic renal failure,* is loss of at least 90 percent of kidney function. The kidneys can't perform their primary function — waste removal. Thus, waste and excess fluid (that would normally be passed through the urethra and out of the body) builds up within the body. To continue living, the patient requires a kidney transplant or dialysis.

High blood pressure, diabetes, and many other conditions that destroy the kidney's filtering mechanism can lead to ESRD. However, individuals who are losing their kidney function are usually unaware of it until they begin to feel sick, and often, they don't start to feel sick until 90 percent of their kidneys' ability to get rid of toxins fails. Before that, with about 70 percent of kidney function lost, high blood pressure, anemia, and bone disease can occur. But still, the individual may be unaware of these abnormalities.

Although efforts to reduce high blood pressure have paid huge dividends, such as a reduction in the rate of heart disease and brain attacks, this isn't true for ESRD. This is probably because, throughout the world, high blood pressure isn't being controlled sufficiently and for long enough.

Whether high blood pressure is untreated or inadequately treated, the result is much the same: ESRD if the patient hasn't already died of heart disease or a brain attack.

Currently, around 506,000 people in the United States are being treated for ESRD and the number rises 10 percent each year. About half of those with ESRD are men. About two-thirds are Caucasian, and about one-third of the population is African American. The largest group is between 45 and 64 years of age. Almost a quarter of those with ESRD die each year. The cost of caring for them is 16 billion dollars each year.

The most common reason for ESRD is currently diabetes (33 percent of the time). The second most common cause is high blood pressure (25 percent of the time). Internal diseases of the kidney account for the rest.

The person with untreated ESRD is very ill. Symptoms affect the entire body and include the following:

- ✔ Fatigue and weakness
- ✔ Easy bruising
- ✔ Itchy skin
- ✔ A metallic taste in the mouth

- ✔ Breath that smells of urine
- ✔ Shortness of breath (even while sitting still and more with minimal activity)
- ✔ Nausea and vomiting
- ✔ Impotency
- ✔ Frequent urination that interrupts sleep
- ✔ Cramping and spasms in the legs (especially at night while trying to sleep)
- ✔ Irritability
- ✔ Unconsciousness

These signs and symptoms subside after treatment begins. Whether the kidneys fail because of high blood pressure, diabetes, or some other cause, the treatment at that stage, as far as the kidneys are concerned, is the same: dialysis or kidney transplantation.

Understanding the Causes of Brain Attacks

Annually, at least 140,000 people die from brain attacks (the term I prefer over "stroke" because it's similar to a "heart attack"), and 650,000 more survive it in the United States. But brain attack survivors may live out the rest of their lives as dependents — unable to speak coherently and/or confined to a wheelchair because of the paralysis that results. There are 6.5 million such people alive in the United States.

The belief that brain attacks were random events, like bolts of lightning, persisted into the twentieth century along with the term *apoplexy,* coming from a Greek word meaning "to be thunderstruck." Apoplexy was the word that folks used back then to refer to a brain attack. Considered unpreventable, a brain attack was thought of as an accident, which explains the term *cerebrovascular accident.* This is clearly not the case, however, as you'll discover.

 Brain attacks, perhaps more than heart attacks and kidney failure, are preventable.

Progress in the treatment of high blood pressure between 1960 and 1990 made this complication of high blood pressure less common. More recently, however, the prevention of brain attacks has slowed down. Even with the reduction in the incidence of brain attacks, it remains the third leading cause of death after heart attacks and cancer.

Although the correlation between high blood pressure and brain attacks is unmistakable, brain attacks can come about in a variety of ways. Brain attacks can result from atherosclerosis, a cerebral embolus, or a brain hemorrhage.

High blood pressure

 High blood pressure is the most important factor in the development of a brain attack, and its control can prevent such an attack. High blood pressure may hasten a brain attack by

✔ Speeding up the development of atherosclerosis

✔ Promoting the thickening of the middle layer of the arteries, thus causing narrowing of the arteries and reduced blood flow into the brain

✔ Damaging small arteries to the point that they collapse

✔ Increasing the size of an aneurysm in the brain

✔ Causing thinning of the aneurysm to the point of rupture and hemorrhage

✔ Causing formation of the aneurysms in the subarachnoid space that rupture to produce a subarachnoid hemorrhage

Many clinical trials have shown that reduction of blood pressure reduces the incidence of brain attacks, no matter how high the initial blood pressure or how old the patient. All types of brain attacks are reduced, from those caused by clots to those caused by hemorrhage.

Atherosclerosis

Just as *atherosclerosis* (damage to the inside of arteries caused by cholesterol deposits) can affect the arteries of the heart, it can also affect the arteries leading into and within the brain. About 60 percent of all brain attacks result from *atherosclerosis,* which is characterized by fatty deposits on the inner walls of the arteries. As a result, blood flow to critical parts of the brain is diminished. If the blood flow ceases entirely, a brain attack may occur.

The blood supply to the brain has multiple sources. Left and right arteries (cerebral arteries) entering the skull in the front of the brain combine with left and right vertebral arteries entering the skull in the back of the brain to produce a circle of blood supply called the *circle of Willis* at the base of the brain. If one of the arteries is blocked, blood from the other arteries can fill the circle and provide blood to all areas of the brain. So if one fails, another artery may provide the needed blood. But when several sources of blood are blocked, the brain tissue dies if the circulation isn't reopened within three hours.

Cerebral embolus

Approximately 25 percent of brain attacks are due to cerebral emboli. A *cerebral embolus* is a blood clot (a solid mass of blood cells, protein, and other blood substances) or solid tissue broken off from an *atherosclerotic plaque* (an irregularity inside the artery that's the end result of a cholesterol deposit) that travels into the brain. The bloodstream carries the atherosclerotic plaque particle from its site of origin, often a large artery in the neck, into the arteries of the brain where it becomes wedged and cuts off circulation.

Blood clots usually come from the left atrium of the heart in the following manner: When the heart loses its regular beating pattern and gives way to uncoordinated twitching movements called *atrial fibrillation,* the heart's chamber (the left atrium) fails to empty out the blood that's in it completely; then the pool of blood that remains forms clots that can break off and travel via the bloodstream into the arteries of the brain.

Brain hemorrhage

Brain hemorrhage — bleeding within the brain or between the skull and the brain — accounts for the other 15 percent of brain attacks. Two-thirds of brain hemorrhages occur within the brain, and a third of brain hemorrhages occur outside the brain in the *subarachnoid space* — the technical term for the thin separation between the inside of your bony skull and the outside of your brain's fleshy gray matter.

As a result of high blood pressure or other diseases that weaken the muscular wall of the artery, one or more little pouches called an *aneurysm* may form in artery wall. With the appearance of a balloon attached to the artery, these aneurysms can burst and bleed into the brain. The brain doesn't have extra space to make room for the extra blood. Bleeding within the brain can also occur as a result of trauma to the head.

Bleeding within the subarachnoid space is usually from an aneurysm that forms inside the skull but outside the brain. If it ruptures, the blood flows around the brain, causing increased pressure and a severe headache that's often accompanied by vomiting.

Chapter 4

Eating and High Blood Pressure

● ●

In This Chapter
▶ Following a diet that lowers blood pressure
▶ Finding out how DASH can help
▶ Lowering salt intake and losing weight, too
▶ Watching your kilocalories and seeking assistance
▶ Cutting back on salt

● ●

*T*hey say that you are what you eat. When it comes to blood pressure, that statement is truer than you may realize. Weight loss with the help of a well-balanced diet and salt intake reduction can lower blood pressure. These approaches, however, haven't successfully lowered blood pressure permanently and kept it down in most patients. A new approach is needed.

In this chapter, you discover a new approach to healthy eating — the DASH diet. I explain how you can use it to reduce your blood pressure, no matter what your blood pressure level is now. For those of you who want to reduce your weight, I provide a sensible, balanced program to help you get there. I try not to use the D (diet) word, but I encourage you to follow a sensible nutritional program.

DASHing Down Your Blood Pressure

Based on the results of studies at four major medical centers in the United States, the "Dietary Approach to Stop Hypertension" (DASH), was published in the *New England Journal of Medicine* (April 1997). All patients on the DASH diet successfully reduced their systolic and diastolic blood pressure.

This was achieved without special foods, food supplements, drugs, and without weekly meetings. Furthermore, it was achieved without emphasizing weight loss by reducing kilocalories, without insisting on salt intake reduction, and without demanding exercise.

Creation of the DASH began when researchers noted that vegetarians generally have lower blood pressure and a lower incidence of coronary heart disease and brain attacks than nonvegetarians. Exactly why this was so wasn't clear. The big difference between vegetarians and nonvegetarians is that the former eat more fruits and vegetables than the latter. They also, of course, eat no meat and generally have less cholesterol and saturated fat in their pattern of eating.

A vegetarian program isn't practical as a recommendation for the American public, so scientists attempted to recreate the vegetarian program while permitting some meat.

Getting with the program

The DASH program is usually based on a 2,000-kilocalorie-a-day diet. If you need fewer kilocalories to maintain your weight, you should take the lower number of servings. If you need more kilocalories, take the higher number of servings.

If you find that following DASH is too difficult, don't hesitate to ask your doctor for a referral to a dietitian.

The 2,000 kilocalorie DASH eating plan has the following foods and servings:

✔ 7 to 8 servings of grains and grain products daily

A serving is 1 slice of bread, ½ bagel, ½ cup dry cereal, ½ cup cooked rice, pasta, or other cereal

✔ 4 to 5 servings of vegetables daily

A serving is 1 cup of raw leafy vegetables, ½ cup cooked vegetables, 6 ounces vegetable juice

✔ 4 to 5 servings of fruit daily

A serving is 6 ounces of fruit juice, 1 medium fruit, ½ cup dried fruit, ½ cup of fresh, frozen, or canned fruit

✔ 2 to 3 servings of low-fat or nonfat dairy products daily

A serving is 1 cup 1 percent milk, 1 cup low-fat yogurt, and 1.5 ounces nonfat cheese

✔ 2 or fewer servings of meats, poultry, or fish daily

A serving is 3 ounces of cooked lean meat, fish, or poultry

✔ 2½ servings of fats

A serving is 1 tsp oil, butter, margarine, mayonnaise, or 1 tbsp regular or 2 tbsp light salad dressing

✔ 4 to 5 servings of nuts, seeds, or legumes per week

A serving is ⅓ cup nuts, 2 tablespoons seeds, ½ cup cooked legumes, or 3 ounces tofu

✔ **5 servings of sweets per week including 1 tbsp sugar, 1 tbsp jelly or jam, ½ ounce jelly beans, or 8 ounces of lemonade**

Examples of good food choices in each group include

✔ **Grains and grain products:** Whole wheat breads, English muffins, pita bread, high-fiber cereals, and oatmeal

✔ **Vegetables:** Tomatoes, potatoes, carrots, peas, squash, broccoli, turnip greens, collards, kale, spinach, artichokes, green beans, and sweet potatoes

✔ **Fruits:** Apples, apricots, bananas, dates, grapes, oranges, orange juice, grapefruit, grapefruit juice, mangos, melons, peaches, pineapples, prunes, raisins, strawberries, and tangerines

✔ **Dairy products:** Skim or 1 percent milk, skim or low-fat buttermilk, nonfat or low-fat yogurt, part-skim mozzarella cheese and nonfat cheese

✔ **Meats, poultry, and fish:** Lean meats, poultry without skin, and no frying or sautéing

✔ **Nuts, seeds, and legumes:** Almonds, mixed nuts, peanuts, peanut butter, walnuts, sesame or sunflower seeds, kidney beans, pinto beans, navy beans, lentils, split peas, garbanzo beans, and tofu

To make up your daily nutrition, Table 4-1 shows a sample menu from which you can fill in the blanks.

Table 4-1	2,000 kilocalorie DASH menu		
Breakfast	*Lunch*	*Dinner*	*Snack*
2 grains	1 meat	1 meat	1 fruit
1 dairy	1 dairy	3 grains	1 grain

Breakfast	Lunch	Dinner	Snack
2 fruits	1 grain	2 vegetables	1 nuts
1 grain	1 fat	1 vegetable	
1 fat	1 vegetable	1½ fat servings	
	1 fruit	1 fruit	

As you follow this diet you can make it easier for yourself in a variety of ways:

✔ Don't try to change all at once. Gradually reduce your meats and increase your fruits and vegetables.

✔ Make it easier to increase fruit and vegetable servings by having two at each meal and two for a snack.

✔ If you're lactose intolerant, take lactase pills with the dairy foods or buy lactose-free milk.

✔ Use the percent Daily Values on food labels to pick the foods that are lowest in saturated fats, total fats, cholesterol, and salt.

✔ Reduce your fats so that you're eating half as much and emphasize vegetable over animal fats.

✔ Avoid soda, alcohol, and other sugar-sweetened drinks.

✔ Use fruits as desserts.

✔ Make grains, such as pasta and rice or beans and vegetables, the center of the meal rather than meat, fish, or poultry.

Slimming Down to Lower Your Blood Pressure

The fatter you are, the higher your blood pressure. More than 50 percent of the population is now overweight or obese as defined by the body mass index (BMI). In this section, you can discover how to calculate your BMI. You can find out whether your weight falls within the range of acceptable weights for your height, and you find out how to calculate the number of kilocalories you need to lose weight if you are heavy or maintain a normal weight if not.

Weighing in

In order to use weight loss to lower your blood pressure, you need to know what your ideal weight should be. If you're already within the correct range of weights for your height, it's not likely that further weight loss can lower your blood pressure much more. If you're overweight or obese, weight loss to your ideal range significantly lowers your blood pressure.

Based on studies of many healthy men and women, your ideal weight range can be determined in the following manner:

✔ If you're a woman, give yourself 100 pounds for being 5 feet tall and add 5 pounds for every inch over 5 feet. For example, if you're 5 feet 3 inches, your appropriate weight is 115 pounds. The appropriate range is that weight plus or minus 10 percent. The appropriate range for a woman who is 5 feet 3 inches tall would be 104 to 126 pounds.

✔ If you're a man, give yourself 106 pounds for being 5 feet tall and 6 pounds more for every inch over 5 feet. A 5-foot-6-inch male should weigh about 142 pounds. The appropriate weight range is then 128 to 156 pounds.

You can also use your BMI to find out if you're under or overweight. The BMI is a number that takes into account your height to determine whether your weight is too high. This is only fair. A 5-foot-4-inch woman who weighs 150 pounds is overweight but a 5-foot-9-inch woman who weighs the same isn't overweight.

If you're good at math (or good with a calculator), you can determine your BMI for yourself. Take your weight in pounds and multiply it by 705. Divide the result by your height in inches. Divide that result by your height in inches again. This is your body mass index in meters per kilogram squared. (Transferring pounds and inches into kilograms and meters is accomplished by the 705-fudge factor.)

By definition, a BMI of 25 to 29.9 is an overweight BMI, and a BMI of 30 or greater is obese. A BMI of 19 to 25 is normal in weight.

So, for example, a 150-pound woman with a height of 5 feet and 4 inches or 64 inches is overweight with a BMI of 27.5. A 150-pound woman with a height of 5 feet and 9 inches or 69 inches has a normal BMI of 22.2.

Determining your daily caloric needs

Caloric needs are different for different ages, sexes, and levels of activity. For example, if a woman is pregnant or breastfeeding, she obviously needs more kilocalories. If a person is trying to lose weight, then reducing the total kilocalories per day can accomplish this. After you know your appropriate weight for your height, you can determine the number of kilocalories that you require each day to maintain that weight as well as the reduction in kilocalories that can result in weight loss. This may best be done with a dietitian to make sure you're getting the right nutrients while staying within your daily caloric limits.

A pound of fat contains 3,500 kilocalories. To lose a pound of fat, therefore, you must eat 3,500 kilocalories less than you need. You can do this by a daily reduction of 500 kilocalories for seven days or by doing 200 kilocalories of exercise a day and reducing the diet by only 300 kilocalories daily. For most people, a combination of diet and exercise works much better than diet alone.

You don't have to lose weight all the way down to your appropriate range to benefit from weight loss. A loss of 5 to 10 percent of your current weight brings important benefits in terms of blood pressure, blood fats, and blood glucose if diabetes is present.

Imagine, for example, a 5-foot-3-inch woman who weighs 150 pounds. Her appropriate weight is 115 pounds within a range of 104 to 126 pounds.

If this woman weighed 115 pounds, she would require 115×10 or 1,150 kilocalories plus more depending on her level of exercise. If she is sedentary, she's entitled to 10 percent more kilocalories for a total of about 1,265 kilocalories daily. If she is moderately active, she gets 20 percent more for a total of 1,380 kilocalories daily. A very active woman may need 40 percent or more extra kilocalories to cover her exercise needs. This would take her up to 1,610 kilocalories. By reducing her daily intake to 1,400 while doing 300 kilocalories of exercise daily, she will lose a pound of fat a week.

After you have the total kilocalories, you can go back to the DASH program and subtract or add servings appropriately.

Trying Other Diets

Sometimes you need a boost to get you going in the right direction towards weight loss and the resulting reduction in blood pressure. I don't insist that my patients follow a balanced nutrition plan all the time as long as I'm certain that they're generally getting the good nutrition they need. A special plan may be what you need to get you started, and then you can continue on a healthy, balanced program, such as DASH. For example, one of my patients eats nothing but rice and water one week a month, eating balanced meals the rest of the time. He has lost a significant amount of weight, come off all blood pressure medication, and has a blood pressure anyone would envy.

Weight loss is difficult for many reasons. In my experience, most patients do well initially but tend to return to old habits. Still, losing weight and keeping it off is definitely possible. At one time, it was calculated that only one out of twenty people who lost weight would keep it off. Now the figure is closer to one in five.

Successfully losing weight and maintaining it also requires a willingness to exercise. Chapter 6 is all about exercise both for health and for weight loss. If, for some reason, you can't move your legs to exercise, you can get a satisfactory workout using your upper body. When people who are successful at weight loss maintenance are questioned, most of them describe exercise as a key part of their success.

The diets I describe aren't balanced diets and shouldn't be your nutritional plan for more than several weeks to get you going. They're generally associated with regaining the weight if they become your primary program. They're usually boring, repetitious, and have little to do with the pleasure of eating.

- ✔ **Very-low-kilocalorie diets:** These diets provide 400 to 800 kilocalories a day of protein and carbohydrate with supplemental vitamins and minerals. They're safe when supervised by a physician and used when you need rapid weight loss, such as in the case of a heart condition. They result in rapid initial weight loss with a fall in the need for medication for high blood pressure. In fact, if you continue your medication, you may suffer dizziness.

- ✔ **Animal-protein diets** (such as the Atkins diet): Food is limited to animal protein in an effort to maintain body protein, along with vitamins and minerals. Patients often complain of hair loss. Weight is rapidly regained when the diet is discontinued. This isn't a balanced diet.

- ✔ **Fasts:** A fast means giving up all food for a period of time and taking only water and vitamins and minerals. A fast is such a drastic change from normal eating habits that most patients do not remain on the fast for very long and weight is regained.

Using Outside Help

The dietitian can be a tremendous source of information on all aspects of nutrition. He can help you determine your correct weight and how many kilocalories per day you need to reach that weight.

Characteristics of successful losers

What is it about the people who've lost weight and kept it off that's different from you or me, or perhaps just me? The National Weight Loss Registry set out to find out how they do it. They surveyed more than 3,000 people who've lost at least 30 pounds and have kept it off for at least one year.

The people had a starting BMI of 36 and currently have a BMI of 25 on average. They lost an average of 71 pounds. Here are some of their characteristics:

- ✔ 74 percent had at least one overweight parent.

- ✔ 20 percent were overweight by age 18.

- ✔ They had recycled (gained and lost) an average of 271 pounds over their lifetime.

- ✔ Most had lost weight in the usual ways, by restricting foods, portion control, counting kilocalories and limiting fats.

- ✔ Their average kilocalorie intake was 1,400 kilocalories per day.

- ✔ Their average weekly kilocalorie expenditure from exercise was 2,800 kilocalories.

- ✔ 55 percent used a program such as Weight Watchers, Overeaters Anonymous, or a dietitian.

- ✔ 45 percent lost weight on their own.

- ✔ 77 percent reported a medical or emotional trigger causing them to finally lose weight successfully.

If you study these characteristics, you find that these people aren't doing strange things to lose weight. They're using ordinary nutritional plans that are usually balanced along with exercise and sometimes outside help.

Other programs have also proved to be valuable for some people. Many of these programs provide all the food that you care to eat, making it exceedingly easy to follow them (although they can also be exceedingly expensive). These programs emphasize gradual weight loss and a connection to more normal eating habits, both of which seem to be a more successful way to lose weight.

- ✔ **Jenny Craig:** This organization provides the food that you eat, which you must pay for. It offers information on food behavior modification.

- ✔ **Weight Watchers:** This organization emphasizes slow weight loss, exercise, and behavior modification. It charges for weekly attendance at its meetings, which you can find all over the world. It doesn't require that you purchase any products. Foods are available for purchase. It has developed a point program that allows you to eat what you want so long as the total is within the points that you're allowed each day. After you reach your goal weight, you can belong for free as long as you stay at that weight or near it. Weight Watchers is very motivating.

Making the Connection between Salt and High Blood Pressure

Salt, which is made up of 40 percent sodium and 60 percent chloride, is critical to your life. You can't live without it. Sodium helps to maintain your blood's water content, serves to balance the acids and bases in your blood, and is necessary for the movement of electrical charges in the nerves that move our muscles.

It's generally believed that the inability of your kidney to excrete salt is responsible for salt-induced high blood pressure. By increasing blood pressure, more salt is filtered by the kidney and enters the urine, and the body compensates for its inability to excrete salt. This increased blood pressure helps to eliminate more salt, but it also puts a strain on your arteries and sets the downward spiral of blood-pressure damage in motion — a vicious cycle.

The recommendation for salt in the Dietary Guidelines for Americans from the U.S. Department of Health and Human Services as well as the American Heart Association is 2,400 milligrams (mg) daily for adults. This is the amount in 1 teaspoon of salt. The average American consumes 5,000 mg of salt daily — twice the necessary amount. Normal salt balance can be maintained with 500 mg daily (or a little more than one-fourth teaspoon of salt), so Americans are eating ten times as much as they really need.

Surprisingly, you're responsible for only 15 percent of the salt in your diet. Food has about 10 percent of your salt already naturally in it. The food industry is responsible for adding 75 percent of the salt that you consume each day to the prepared foods that you buy.

The only way that you can successfully reduce the salt in your diet is by switching from processed foods to fresh foods or selecting low-salt processed foods.

Buying low-salt foods

The Food and Drug Administration has definite guidelines as to the terms a food company can use when describing the salt in the food on the label. Keep these terms in mind and make a point of buying low-salt foods on your next trip to the grocery store:

- **Sodium free** means less than 5 mg sodium in a portion.

- **Very low sodium** means less than 35 mg sodium in a portion.

- **Low sodium** means less than 140 mg sodium in a portion.

- **Reduced sodium** food contains 25 percent less sodium than the original food item.

- **Light in sodium** food has 50 percent less sodium than the original food item.

- **Unsalted, No salt added,** or **Without added salt** means absolutely no salt has been added to a food that's normally processed with salt.

 Take time to read the Nutrition Facts label on food items. Avoid items that contain more than 180 milligrams of sodium.

Going on a low-salt diet

Besides avoiding high-salt foods, you can make a few other changes to lower your salt intake:

- Cook with herbs, spices, fruit juices, and vinegars for flavor rather than salt.

- Eat fresh vegetables.

- Keep the saltshaker in the kitchen cupboard rather than at the table, where it's so easy to use.

- Use less salt than the recipe calls for.

- Select low-salt canned foods or rinse your food with water.

- Select low-salt frozen dinners.

- Use high-salt condiments, such as ketchup and mustard, sparingly.

✓ Snack on fresh fruits rather than salted crackers or chips.

✓ When eating out, ask that your food be prepared with only a little salt. Request your salad dressing "on the side" of the salad, so you can control the amount that goes on it.

Be careful of salt substitutes. Some contain sodium. Check the label. You could end up eating so much of the substitute in an attempt to get that salty taste that your total sodium intake is just as high as using salt.

Go to www.nhlbi.nih.gov/health/public/ heart/hbp/dash/new_dash.pdf to download the government's "Guide to Lowering Blood Pressure with DASH." You'll find recipes for two levels of salt — 2,300 milligrams a day and 1,500 milligrams a day. You'll also find a lot of help in following this excellent plan to lower blood pressure.

Chapter 5

Avoiding Poison: Tobacco, Alcohol, and Caffeine

. . . .

In This Chapter

▶ Battling bad habits: Contributors to high blood pressure

▶ Quitting tobacco decreases risks

▶ Drowning in alcohol and how it affects your blood pressure

▶ Increasing your blood pressure with caffeine

. . . .

*N*othing you could ever do for your health can make a greater difference than cutting out tobacco, alcohol, and caffeine.

In this chapter, I take up each one of these dangerous habits individually and discuss how they affect your blood pressure. I also discuss how eliminating these poisons from your life can help lower your blood pressure and make your mind and body healthier.

Tobacco, alcohol, and caffeine represent a triple threat to your health. But within that triple threat may also be triple salvation. Reducing or eliminating one of these three poisons often leads to a reduction or elimination of one or both of the others. The tendency to have that cigarette with your scotch or your coffee is eliminated if you don't drink the scotch or the coffee.

Playing with Fire

When you play with fire, you get burned. When you smoke, you run the risk of getting burned inside and out. Whether tobacco is smoked or chewed or taken in by any other means, the nicotine in the tobacco raises the blood pressure. The more you smoke, the higher the nicotine level is in your blood, and the higher your blood pressure. This accounts to a large extent for the great increase in brain attacks (see Chapter 3), heart attacks and pain in the legs due to poor circulation in smokers, sometimes leading to amputation.

Nicotine raises your blood pressure by constricting your blood vessels. This occurs because the oxygen in your blood decreases and because nicotine directly stimulates the production of a hormone, *epinephrine* (also known as adrenaline), in the adrenal gland. Epinephrine raises blood pressure. After tobacco use raises blood pressure, you're at risk of all the medical consequences of high blood pressure (described in Chapter 3), not to mention diseases associated with smoking, such as mouth and lung cancer.

Numerous studies have shown that smoking or chewing tobacco raises blood pressure and that when you stop using tobacco products, your blood pressure falls.

Putting one foot in the grave

Blood pressure elevation is just one of smoking's many consequences. Other smoking-related complications are as follows.

- ✔ Lung cancer is 20 times more likely among smokers than nonsmokers.

- ✔ Cancers of the mouth and throat as well as the bladder are more likely among smokers. The connection isn't as clear, but smoking is also likely to increase the possibility of cancers of the liver, large intestine, pancreas, kidney, and the cervix in women.

- ✔ Coronary heart disease is much more common among smokers, whether they have increased blood pressure or not.

- ✔ Brain attacks (see Chapter 3) are more common among smokers — again, regardless of elevated blood pressure.

- ✔ Bleeding from rupture of the large blood vessel in the abdomen is more common.

- ✔ Chronic lung disease is most often the result of smoking.

- ✔ Lung growth rate is reduced among adolescents who smoke.

- ✔ Women who smoke have trouble conceiving a baby, and if they do, they're more likely to miscarry. Women who smoke also tend to start menopause at a younger age.

- ✔ Smoking reduces bone density and increases the risk of fractures in older women especially.

- ✔ A correlation exists between smoking and depression.

Regarding smokeless tobacco

Smokeless tobacco is tobacco that you chew or put into your nostrils. Types of smokeless tobacco include snuff, which is placed between the cheek and the gum in the United States and is sniffed into the nose in Europe, and chewing tobacco, which is a wad of tobacco that is placed inside the cheek and chewed on to extract the juices. In the process of using either one, a great deal of saliva is produced forcing the user to spit frequently. Not a pretty picture.

Smokeless tobacco provides at least twice as much nicotine as a cigarette. Eight to ten chews a day is equivalent to 40 cigarettes a day in nicotine content. Therefore, using smokeless tobacco damages the heart and blood vessels over the long term, and the effect on the blood pressure is that much greater and of a longer duration. In addition, smokeless tobacco is filled with agents that cause cancer.

Smokeless tobacco won't help you quit smoking. Actually, smokeless tobacco is just as addictive as cigarettes. So don't think that using smokeless tobacco instead of cigarettes can get rid of your nicotine cravings. Instead, smokeless tobacco discolors your teeth, sours your breath, and creates cancer in your throat, voice box, and esophagus.

Everything to gain; nothing to lose

Why should you give up something that you find pleasurable and that may even make it easier to keep those extra pounds off? As far as the pounds, you can get rid of those with more exercise and fewer kilocalories. As for the pleasure, the short and long-term health consequences when you quit are as follows:

✔ The healing starts within 12 hours as the carbon monoxide levels in your body fall and your heart and lungs begin to function more normally with a resultant fall in your blood pressure and your heart rate.

✔ Your taste buds and your sense of smell return in a few days.

✔ Your face wrinkles far less as you age.

✔ If you're attempting to get pregnant, achieving pregnancy is easier; and after you're pregnant, the pregnancy proceeds in a healthier manner.

✔ Your smoker's cough diminishes after a few days, though it may last for a while as your rejuvenated lungs begin to mobilize and expel the gunk accumulated over years of smoking.

✔ The stench of stale smoke and the mess of cigarette butts will be gone along with the expense of smoking and the time wasted buying cigarettes and finding a place to smoke away from others.

✔ Your risk of early death is the same as that of a nonsmoker after 10 to 15 years of no cigarettes, depending on how long you smoked.

✔ After five years, the risk of cancer of the mouth and throat along with bladder cancer and cancer of the cervix in women is significantly diminished.

✔ After ten years, you have half the chance of developing lung cancer than if you continued to smoke.

The time that you add onto your life can't be totaled up in terms of just days but productive, healthy days — days that you otherwise may have spent gasping for breath with an oxygen tube in your nose, too short of breath to walk over to your grandchild and hug her.

Kicking the habit

The past few years have seen a smoking-cessation-treatment revolution. Nicotine gum followed what began as psychotherapy. Then came nicotine patches, and now drugs that don't contain nicotine take away the craving for nicotine. In this section, you can find something that appeals to you.

No one way works for all people. Try each one. If it doesn't work for you, try another technique. Something will click eventually.

You benefit from stopping smoking no matter what your age or physical condition.

Follow these steps and your success is far more likely:

1. **Prepare yourself.**

   Set a quit date and make it special. After all, your body is being reborn. It will be a day of celebration for the rest of your life.

   Make a list of reasons to quit. Improve your fitness, which makes any significant change easier to manage. Avoid drinks with caffeine to help you to sleep after you quit smoking. Satisfy your hunger with low-calorie beverages or snacks. Relax yourself by exercising, taking a bath, or meditation. Treat any cough with cough drops or hard candy.

2. **Benefit from the support of friends and loved ones.**

   Let everyone know you're quitting and ask for help, especially by not smoking in your presence. Even better, ask them to stop with you. Use individual or group counseling to support you. This may mean talking to someone as many as several times a day as you're trying to quit. Check with your doctor or other healthcare provider for ideas that she may have to help you.

3. **Find distractions that substitute for the urge to smoke.**

   Stop activities that you combine with smoking, such as drinking alcohol or coffee, the morning break, or whatever you know to be a smoking trigger. Change your routine to emphasize the lifestyle change. Find an enjoyable substitute for smoking. Switch to a brand that you don't like that's low nicotine before you stop. Smoke only half the cigarette. Limit yourself to an increasingly smaller fixed number of cigarettes daily. After you get down to seven or less, set a quit date. Drink plenty of noncaloric fluids, such as water.

4. **Make use of the medications that have proven to be effective in helping a person quit.**

   Ask your doctor about nicotine replacement therapy and smoking cessation aids.

5. **Prepare for relapses.**

   Everyone who has successfully quit smoking has probably done it on the second, third, or fourth try. Giving yourself another chance to succeed if things go wrong temporarily is essential. If you relapse, it usually occurs within the first three months.

 Should you relapse, begin the process of quitting again as soon as possible. The less you smoke, the easier it will be to quit again. Try to recognize the situations that blocked your success and avoid them the next time around.

Two effective methods for quitting smoking are nicotine replacement therapy and smoking cessation aids. Some methods can be bought over the counter while others require a prescription from your doctor. The details of each method are provided as follows:

✔ **Nicotine-replacement therapy:** The point of nicotine replacement therapy is to deliver small doses of nicotine (through gum, patches, inhalers, or nasal sprays) to avoid withdrawal from tobacco. If you have high blood pressure associated with nicotine intake, you want to use nicotine replacement therapy as short a time as possible because nicotine in this form raises your blood pressure.

✔ **Smoking-cessation aids:** Bupropion SR, tradename Zyban, acts to disrupt the addictive power of nicotine. At a dose of 300 mg, given as 150 mg twice daily, available by prescription, it has proved its effectiveness in large studies of smokers.

A combination of bupropion and a nicotine-replacement aid accomplished a much higher rate of quitting than either one did alone.

Tapping into resources

With the availability of the Internet, you have many resources to help you quit smoking at the peck of a key on your computer keyboard. If you're computer-challenged, you can access these resources by mail or telephone. Here are the best of the lot:

✔ The National Institutes of Health contains the **National Cancer Institute** (NCI). The NCI does research on quitting smoking, promotes programs to decrease the impact of smoking on health, and publishes materials on the Internet and in hard copy with tips on quitting and avoiding secondhand smoke. The NCI supports the Cancer Information Service from which these materials are available at 1-800-4-Cancer. The Web address is http://cis.nci.nih.gov.

✔ **The National Institute on Drug Abuse** (NIDA) is another part of the National Institutes of Health. It supports research on cigarettes and other sources of nicotine as an addictive drug. Fact sheets are available concerning drug abuse and addition at 1-888-NIH-NIDA. The Web address is www.health.org.

✔ **The Office on Smoking and Health National Center for Chronic Disease Prevention** has a database of smoking and health-related materials at 1-800-232-1311 or on the Web at www.cdc.gov/tobacco.

✔ **The Agency for Healthcare Research and Quality** has smoking cessation guidelines and other materials for both physicians and the public at 1-800-358-9295 or on the Web at www.ahcpr.gov.

✔ **The American Cancer Society** has many pamphlets and Web pages on quitting smoking as well as a bibliography of books and tapes on quitting at 1-800-227-2345 or www.cancer.org.

✔ **The American Lung Association** has both information and clinics to help you stop smoking at 1-800-586-4872 or www.lungusa.org.

✔ **The American Heart Association** provides information on smoking-cessation programs in schools, workplaces, and healthcare sites. To obtain, call 1-800-242-8721 or visit the Internet at www.americanheart.org.

✔ **Nicotine Anonymous** is a 12-step program. To find out more, call 1-415-750-0328 or visit the Internet at www.nicotine-anonymous.org.

Relating Alcohol to High Blood Pressure

This section tackles the second-most lethal thing that you can put into your body: alcohol. Or maybe it's the *most* lethal. I guess it depends on whether you specialize in lungs or livers. (In this section, I'm addressing people who drink more than a glass or two of wine a day and more than ten glasses a week.)

Alcohol raises blood pressure. Comparing the blood pressure of heavy drinkers (men who drink more than ten and women who drink more than five alcoholic beverages per week) with moderate drinkers and those who don't drink, shows that alcohol does indeed raise blood pressure. When nondrinkers drink alcohol, their blood pressure rises, and when heavy drinkers stop drinking, their blood pressure falls.

Abruptly stopping alcohol may cause a rise in blood pressure, so a doctor must monitor this carefully.

Drinking large quantities of alcohol in one sitting also raises blood pressure, but it returns to normal if the drinking doesn't continue. However, an individual who drinks excessively for extended periods of time has a persistent increase in blood pressure. The longer a person drinks, the higher the blood pressure.

It doesn't hurt to reemphasize that stopping one bad habit may ease the stopping of another. Cigarettes and alcohol go together like Fred Astaire and Ginger Rogers, but smoking and drinking isn't graceful or charming. Between 80 to 95 percent of alcoholics smoke cigarettes. Eliminating the power of one goes a long way towards eliminating the power of the other.

Considering the effects of alcoholism

Alcoholism, defined as the habitual or compulsive consumption of alcoholic liquor to excess, is an inherited physical abnormality, an inborn condition related to a certain type of body chemistry. Alcoholism is *not* a moral weakness.

A major medical consequence of alcoholism is the occurrence of brain attacks at a much higher rate. A study in *Stroke* (May 1998) showed that drinking four beers or the equivalent on a daily basis led to a considerable increase in brain attacks, even more that the increase in brain attacks caused by heavy smoking (more than 20 cigarettes daily).

If you're taking medication for high blood pressure and drinking heavily at the same time, you need to determine whether you're an alcoholic to clarify the role of your drinking in your blood pressure.

You may be an alcoholic if you answer yes to two or more of the following questions. Have you

- ✔ Tried to reduce your drinking?
- ✔ Felt angry when someone talked to you about your drinking?
- ✔ Felt guilty about drinking?
- ✔ Used alcohol in the morning to "start the day" and settle your nerves?

Another way to determine whether you're an alcoholic is to count the number of drinks that you consume in a week. (A drink is a 12-ounce bottle of beer, 5 ounces of wine, or 1½ ounces of hard liquor.) Alcoholic men usually consume 15 or more drinks per week, and alcoholic women consume 12 or more. Those who consume more than five drinks in one sitting at least once a week are also considered alcoholics. Usually, alcoholics also

- ✔ Crave alcohol.
- ✔ Lose control when they drink.
- ✔ Have withdrawal symptoms if they don't drink.
- ✔ Have a tolerance to alcohol.

Alcohol's other consequences

The following list of health consequences from excessive alcohol use is long. Unfortunately, you don't get one or another of these complications, but all of them at the same time.

- ✔ Depression of the central nervous system with loss of ability to perform complex tasks, such as driving; decreased attention span and short-term memory; impaired motor coordination
- ✔ Degeneration of the brain with loss of coordination and emotional instability, and nerve degeneration with severe pain
- ✔ Addiction to tranquilizers to treat the emotional instability
- ✔ Physical damage in motor-vehicle crashes
- ✔ Increased risk of suicide and homicide
- ✔ Increased risk of unplanned pregnancy and sexually-transmitted diseases
- ✔ Giving birth to a baby with fetal-alcohol syndrome, stunted growth, mental retardation, and other abnormalities of the face and heart
- ✔ Poor nutrition from an irritated liver and intestinal tract, which produces heartburn, nausea, and gas
- ✔ Alcoholic heart disease
- ✔ Loss of sex drive
- ✔ Neglect of food intake and physical appearance

✔ Sleep loss

✔ Severe inflammation of the pancreas with severe abdominal pain and nausea

✔ Cirrhosis of the liver with gastrointestinal bleeding, liver failure, and death

✔ Increased incidence of cancer

The combination of drinking and smoking greatly increases the risk of cancer. A drinker is six times more likely to get mouth and throat cancer as compared to a nondrinker. A smoker is seven times more likely to get mouth and throat cancer as compared to a nonsmoker. But the individual who drinks and smokes is 38 times more likely to have mouth and throat cancer than the individual who neither drinks nor smokes.

Gaining by restraining

All the medical consequences of alcoholism start to reverse after you give up alcohol, particularly, for our purposes, the blood pressure. Cirrhosis of the liver, however, is irreversible after it occurs. In addition, you may regain your job, your family, and other loved ones, and your self-respect.

Through the years, the study of alcoholism and its treatment has proven useful in many ways. First of all, the more help that the alcoholic gets and uses, the greater the chance for prolonged sobriety. Specifically:

✔ Only 4 percent of alcoholics who try quitting on their own are sober after a year.

✔ 50 percent of alcoholics who go through treatment are sober after a year.

✔ 70 percent of alcoholics who go through treatment and regularly attend Alcoholics Anonymous are sober after a year.

✔ 90 percent of alcoholics who go through treatment, attend Alcoholics Anonymous, and go to aftercare once a week are sober after one year.

Treatment and follow-up after treatment is undoubtedly valid and important. Treatment consists of a brief intervention, during which the alcoholic is convinced to undergo therapy to stop drinking, and then a period of total abstinence from alcohol called *detoxification,* followed by techniques that keep the alcoholic sober for the rest of her life. These techniques include drugs and Alcoholics Anonymous.

Total abstinence from alcohol is the goal of treatment. Absolutely no amount of alcohol, no matter how small, is acceptable.

Attending Alcoholics Anonymous

A major step that the alcoholic can take is to join Alcoholics Anonymous (AA). More than 1 million recovered alcoholics are in AA in the United States and another million are in other countries. AA members meet in groups, large and small, to support one another. About 51,000 AA groups meet in the United States, and one can be found near you. Check online at www.alcoholics-anonymous.org or write to the main office to find a support group near you: Alcoholics Anonymous, Grand Central Station, P.O. Box 459, New York, NY 10163.

The support of AA is tremendously helpful for the alcoholic who utilizes it.

Can moderate drinking benefit your health?

For years, people thought that a drink a day would keep the doctor away. And a number of studies have shown that people who drink moderately (no more than two drinks daily for men and one for women) have improvements in the health of their heart and a lower rate of death than people who don't drink at all.

But a more recent study of 5,500 men in Scotland published in the *British Medical Journal* (June 1999) showed that drinking two drinks daily led to a higher risk of dying from all causes as compared with men who drank less alcohol. In another study from Harvard Medical School, a fat increase was discovered in the livers of men who ate well but had a daily dose of alcohol not large enough to cause inebriation. So a word to the wise: Don't start drinking to obtain the medical "benefits" of alcohol.

Locating useful resources

Numerous resources are available to the alcoholic who wishes to recover if only she makes use of them. Some are listed below in no particular order. If you have access, you can find tons of information on the Internet. If not, call the phone number I've added to each resource.

- ✔ **The Internet Alcohol Recovery Center** is a central source for information on every aspect of alcohol abuse and treatment. A service of the University of Pennsylvania Health System, it has links to numerous resources and is a great place to start your education. It has a substance abuse library and a directory of treatment professionals and support groups. You can call them at 215-243-9959 or find them online at www.uphs.upenn.edu/recovery/index. html.

✔ **Alcoholics Anonymous** has numerous sites on the Internet because so many of these groups dot the planet, but the central Web site is www.alcoholics-anonymous.org. Most of the organization's publications are online along with directions to their groups worldwide. This is a key resource for anyone who lives with an alcoholic or is trying to quit alcohol. You can also call them at 212-870-3400.

✔ **The American Council on Alcoholism** is a national nonprofit organization dedicated to addressing alcoholism as a treatable disease. Its Web site has useful links to sites concerning college drinking, drunk driving, general information on alcoholism, government resources, professional organizations that deal with alcoholism, treatment and recovery, drugs that help, and to the Web sites of the alcohol industry. Their site, www.aca-usa.org, answers any question that you may have about alcoholism. You can call them at 800-527-5344.

✔ **Al-Anon/Alateen** provides help for the victims (loved ones?) of the alcoholic. It uses the principles of AA to help these people regain control over their lives and to see what action they can take to help the alcoholic. You find information on meetings, resources, and plenty of other help. Look for them at www.al-anon. alateen.org or call 888-425-2666.

✔ **Mothers Against Drunk Driving** is another nationwide organization that provides information. It has over 600 chapters in this country and is dedicated to finding effective solutions to drunk driving and underage driving. Find them at www.madd.org/madd/aboutus. Their phone number is 800-438-6233.

Getting High on Caffeine

Caffeine is a chemical compound that's found in the leaves, seeds, and fruits of more than 63 plant species but most commonly comes from coffee and cocoa beans, cola nuts, and tea leaves. Coffee isn't the only source of caffeine. A can of cola contains 45 mg. Green tea contains 30 mg of caffeine. An ounce of chocolate has 20 mg in it. Even Anacin comes in at 65 mg for two tablets.

While the case against caffeine isn't nearly as tidy as that against tobacco and alcohol, no matter what form it's taken in, caffeine has been shown to temporarily raise blood pressure. Although a cup or two of coffee doesn't seem to be damaging over the long-term, our current tendency to drink multiple cups of "high octane" (heavily caffeinated) coffee is a definite cause of a persistent elevation in blood pressure.

People who drink four to five cups of coffee daily have an increase in blood pressure of 5 mm Hg. (See Chapter 1 for more on blood pressure measurement.) If they continue to drink the same amount, the blood pressure may fall if they don't have high blood pressure already. If they do, they may be more sensitive to the blood pressure-raising effect of caffeine, and their blood pressure rise is sustained. This is particularly true of the elderly population.

A 5 mm Hg rise in blood pressure may sound trivial, but it results in a 21 percent rise in the incidence of heart disease and a 34 percent increase in the incidence of brain attacks (see Chapter 3). In addition, when combined with alcohol and/or tobacco, which is so often the case, it greatly increases the blood pressure-raising effect of those drugs.

 Having a cup of coffee just before having your blood pressure measured is unwise. The acute elevation in blood pressure may convince your doctor that you have sustained high blood pressure.

An ordinary cup of coffee has 100 mg of caffeine. A tall (12 ounce) cup of coffee at a nice café or fancy coffee shop has 375 mg, while a coffee grande has 550 mg. A short (8 ounce) cup of coffee contains 250 mg. You can see where a few cups of coffee can quickly add up to much more than the recommended maximum of 300 mg.

Caffeine and other health consequences

Caffeine is a mildly addictive drug. When a person stops drinking it, she will have withdrawal symptoms, such as feeling sleepy or overtired or having a severe headache.

Caffeine also has a number of potential medical consequences when taken in large doses (over 300 mg daily) over a period of years:

- Thinning of the bone called *osteoporosis*
- Infertility, birth defects, and miscarriages
- Heartburn (take it from me) and even ulcers due to increased stomach acid production

> ✔ Increased rate of heart disease, if the coffee is unfiltered
>
> ✔ Poor quality sleep and difficulty falling asleep

Caffeine can keep you awake, but it does not improve your performance of complex tasks.

Avoiding the beans, the chocolate, and the soda

If you consume caffeine in the form of no more than two cups of coffee daily, you should have no problem switching to decaffeinated drinks and avoiding other sources of caffeine, such as chocolate. I was in that category when I gave up caffeine, yet I did go through a period of mild withdrawal symptoms.

For the person who takes in much more in the form of giant cups of coffee or many cans of soda daily, the process of quitting caffeine may be more difficult. Here are some practical suggestions:

> ✔ Try to determine how much caffeine you're taking in each day. Check all foods and medications to make sure you're not missing an unexpected source.
>
> ✔ Reduce your intake and see how you feel as you withdraw.
>
> ✔ Gradually reduce your daily caffeine by 50 mg or so until you're free of it.
>
> ✔ Use exercise to give you the energy that you believe was coming from caffeine.
>
> ✔ Avoid the other habits that go with drinking coffee, such as smoking.
>
> ✔ Ask the people you live and eat with to help you by reducing their caffeine intake as well. The improvement they feel will make them grateful.

Using resources

You can check a few Internet sites for the latest information on this controversial drug. Among the best are

- ✔ The Center for Science in the Public Interest is a large Web source of information on exactly what its title suggests. They publish the Nutrition Action Healthletter. As new information on the health effects of caffeine becomes available, you can find it at this site with the address www.cspinet.org. Their phone number is 202-332-9110.

- ✔ Numerous university hospital sites are available on the Internet where you can search for information on caffeine. One of the best is Columbia University's Health Question & Answer Internet Service called "Go Ask Alice." You can find it at www.goaskalice.columbia.edu.

Chapter 6

Exercising Your Way to Lower Blood Pressure

* *

In This Chapter

▶ Understanding why you should exercise

▶ Getting started

▶ Deciding what exercises you like

▶ Knowing your limits

▶ Exercising for weight loss and strength

▶ Moving your body in other ways

* *

*W*hen I see new patients with high blood pressure, I give them a bottle of pills right away. But the pills aren't for oral consumption. They're for dropping on the floor and picking up one at a time several times a day — a good start to an exercise program.

You must make up your mind to exercise. Did you think you were given all those muscles just to cushion your bones? Exercise can lower blood pressure — especially the blood pressure of those who have high blood pressure. The benefits of a regular exercise program can't be denied. Lowering your blood pressure is just one of the many reasons for committing yourself to a regular exercise program. Exercise also causes weight reduction and weight loss maintenance, which also helps to lower blood pressure.

An exercise test can also help find out the people who need to be observed for the development of high blood pressure. Those who have an exaggerated rise in blood pressure during exercise are much more likely to develop sustained high blood pressure later in life. They need to be watched more carefully.

I asked a patient who refused to exercise whether it was because of ignorance or apathy. The patient replied, "I don't know, and I don't care." Read this chapter. Then if you don't exercise, at least it won't be because of ignorance.

Understanding the Benefits of Physical Activity

Exercise strengthens all the muscles that are involved in the movement. If you walk or jog, your leg muscles are strengthened. If you lift packages, your arm muscles are strengthened. Whatever the exercise, your heart muscles are made stronger. At the same time, your body opens up your arteries to allow for more flow of nutrients into the tissues. The combination of a stronger, more efficient heart and more open blood vessels leads to lowering blood pressure.

Lowering your blood pressure is a good enough reason to make exercise an important part of your lifestyle, but if you need more reasons, check out what else exercise can do for you:

- ✔ Improve your memory
- ✔ Reduce the risk of breast cancer and large intestinal cancer

✔ Lower blood sugar, thus protecting you against diabetes

✔ Increase energy level

✔ Improve mood

✔ Make you sexier

✔ Help you sleep better

✔ Strengthen your bones

✔ Lower bad cholesterol and raise good cholesterol

Could you possibly need any more reasons? If you do, pick up a copy of *Fitness For Dummies,* 2nd Edition, by Suzanne Schlosberg and Liz Neporent, MA (Wiley), where you find 100 reasons to become fit.

Preparing for Exercise

You need to take two important steps before you begin an exercise program. First, determine your current physical condition to decide what type of exercise program is right for your current fitness level. Second, choose the exercises that you plan to make part of your program.

Checking your physical condition

Before you start an exercise program, find out the level of your fitness, so that you have something to use to chart your progress. One simple way to test your fitness level is to take your pulse, walk a mile, and note the time that it takes you as well as your pulse rate at the end of the mile. The time and your pulse give you have a baseline.

To take your pulse, place your index and middle finger over the artery in the wrist that's about ½ inch in from the outside of the wrist when it's facing with the palm upward. (Don't use your thumb to feel because it has its own pulse and can confuse your count.) Count the number of beats for 15 seconds and multiply by four to get your one-minute pulse rate. If you can't feel your pulse in the wrist, try feeling the pulse in your neck where it's much stronger. Write down the number before you forget it! You can do this simple test about once a month and you'll be astounded at your progress as your pulse gets slower and slower — indicating a much more efficient heart.

If you haven't exercised for many years, don't start a program without some preparation. If you're over the age of 40, you should talk to your doctor and have a physical examination. Your doctor may recommend an *exercise electrocardiogram,* better known as an exercise test or a stress test. The test looks at the response of your heart to fairly vigorous exercise. If you get through an exercise test without problems such as chest pain, severe shortness of breath, or changes in your electrocardiogram, you're probably in good enough shape to begin an exercise program.

 Ask your doctor to help you map out an exercise plan that can achieve your goal of strengthening your heart and preventing high blood pressure. If you've already been diagnosed with high blood pressure, discuss a plan that can help lower your blood pressure to an agreeable level.

 When you begin your exercise program, start slowly and build up over time. You don't need to rush to get to a certain level of exercise by a certain date. Gradually work your way along until you achieve your goal. You also don't need to go farther and faster after you reach a level of fitness that affects your blood pressure. That desired fitness level may lower your blood pressure by as much as 10 millimeters of mercury systolic (see Chapter 1) — a lowering that's as good as most pills can accomplish. Going farther and faster, however, won't get you much lower than that. If you're really *enjoying* the exercise and *want* to rev it up, that's up to you, but don't think that doing so can further lower your blood pressure.

Choosing exercises

For maximum fitness, most exercise programs combine two types of exercises: aerobic and anaerobic.

- ✔ **Aerobic** means "with oxygen." During aerobic exercise, the body uses oxygen to help provide energy. Aerobic activities can be sustained for more than a few minutes and involve major groups of muscles, particularly the legs but also the arms if you can't use your legs. These activities, such as walking, running, cycling, tennis, basketball, and so forth, get your heart to pump faster during the exercise.

- ✔ **Anaerobic** means "without oxygen." Anaerobic exercises are brief and very intense. They can't be sustained for very long and depend on sources of energy that are already available. Examples are lifting heavy weights and doing the 100-yard dash.

Engaging in a regular aerobic exercise program can, over time, lower your blood pressure up to 10 millimeters of mercury systolic and enable you to get off a blood pressure medication. Anaerobic exercises, although great for increasing the strength of individual muscles, don't go on long enough to improve heart function or lower your blood pressure. But a program of both aerobic and anaerobic exercises gives you the best of both worlds — lower blood pressure and stronger muscles.

The range of aerobic exercise choices is limitless. Mix it up a bit. Play tennis several days a week and do something else, perhaps walking, the other days. Walking is the exercise that almost everybody can do. You don't have to belong to a special club to walk. Unless you live in an area that has snow a good portion of the year, you can walk outside most any day — even in the rain. (Use an umbrella; you won't melt.)

Table 6-1 is a walking program that can get you up to speed eventually but that starts slow enough so that most people can complete the first part without a great deal of difficulty. If the distance is too great for you, begin with half the distance and work your way up until you've accomplished each level once each day for seven days. Don't move to the next level before you've done the previous level seven times.

If you did the test described earlier in this chapter to evaluate your fitness, you already know how fast you can do a mile. Start at that level, not a slower level. If you didn't do a fitness test, begin the seven days at the level that you can do the first time that you try.

Table 6-1 breaks down the walking program into 15 different levels so that you can work your way up to a desired level of fitness to lower your blood pressure. Start at the highest one that you can do now and build from there.

Table 6-1	Walking Program to Achieve Lower Blood Pressure	
Level	*Distance (in miles)*	*Time (in minutes)*
1	1	30
2	1	28
3	1	26
4	1	24
5	1	22
6	1	20
7	1½	32
8	1½	31
9	1½	30
10	1½	29
11	1½	28
12	1½	27
13	1½	26
14	1½	25
15	1½	24

You must complete one level seven times before moving on to the next level.

When you reach the last level, you can stay at that level permanently. You'll have an acceptable workout that'll make a significant difference in your blood pressure as well as other aspects of your health. Surely you can spare less than half an hour daily to make a huge impact on your health.

Walking is great exercise, and certainly one of the simplest, but don't feel like you *have* to walk to enjoy the pressure-lowering effects of exercise. If you prefer to do some other types of aerobic activities, feel free! Just make sure that you choose aerobically effective activities that you're able to do and able to stick with. *What* you do doesn't really matter; you just have to be sure to do *something*.

Knowing How Much to Do

People with high blood pressure have a post-exercise fall in blood pressure that may last seven or eight hours. Therefore, *daily* exercise can have a much more profound effect on your blood pressure than exercise that's done only three or four times a week.

You want to know whether your exercise is making a difference in your fitness. You could do a fitness test each time, but that's not a good idea because you won't make huge strides each time that you exercise, and you'll definitely be disappointed.

Rate your physical activity of choice according to the Perceived Exertion Scale to determine whether the activity is making a difference in your fitness. To use this scale, rate the degree of your exertion while performing a certain activity from being very, very light to being very, very hard — according to your personal physical ability level. In between are very light, fairly light, somewhat hard, hard, and very hard.

If you exercise to the level of very hard, you're doing the amount of exercise that's most beneficial.

Keep in mind that as your fitness level increases, your definition of very hard changes. What was once very hard may become fairly light. Very hard exercise also corresponds to a level at which you start having trouble talking comfortably.

Exercise is beneficial for every stage of high blood pressure. However, doctors generally recommend that people with blood pressure in the higher stages 2 and 3, where the blood pressure is greater than 160 systolic and 100 diastolic, do their exercise at a slightly lower level than stage 1 patients. Referring to the Perceived Exertion Scale, stage 2 and 3 patients should work at a level of "somewhat hard" rather than "very hard."

Exercising to Lose Weight

Exercise can help you lose weight. If you expect to lose weight as you exercise, you need to exercise at least six days a week for at least 30 minutes each time.

A pound of fat contains 3,500 *kilocalories* (kcals). To lose a pound of fat, you must do at least 3,500 kilocalories of exercise greater than the number of kilocalories that you eat. For example, if you eat 2,000 kilocalories each day to maintain your weight, doing 500 kilocalories of exercise daily more than you usually do causes a weight loss of a pound in seven days (500 times 7 equals 3,500). Doing only 250 kilocalories of extra exercise takes 14 days to lose the same pound.

An hour of walking daily, which burns 4 kilocalories per minute, results in 240 kilocalories of energy loss daily.

Exercising for Strength

A complete exercise program includes both aerobic exercises to lower your blood pressure and anaerobic exercises to strengthen your muscles. Strengthening your muscles allows you to do more aerobic exercise as well as improve your balance. To add an anaerobic element to your workout, get yourself some *dumbbells* of various weights and some *barbells,* to which you can add progressively more weight as you get stronger.

If you have high blood pressure, use weight sizes that allow you to do many repetitions of an exercise instead of doing a few extreme lifts with very large weights. Extreme lifting may suddenly raise your blood pressure to unacceptable levels.

A weight lifting program requires no more than 15 minutes of your time about five days a week. Do it for two days, skip a day, for another three days, skip a day, then back to two days, and so on. These breaks allow your muscles to recover between workouts.

The following list describes seven exercises that can improve your upper-body strength. You can do these exercises in 15 minutes. Simply do 15 repetitions of each exercise and move on to the next. Each series of 15 repetitions of seven exercises is called a *circuit.* You should do two circuits without stopping each time that you exercise. Start with an amount of weight that allows you to complete the 15 repetitions. If you can't do 15, you're using too much weight and overexerting yourself.

Evaluating the strength of your upper and lower body

Count how many push-ups you can do to evaluate your upper-body strength. To do a push-up, lie face down on the floor with your palms about shoulder-width apart. Push yourself up off the floor, straightening your arms and keeping your back and legs straight. Lower yourself until your chest just touches the floor, but don't let your weight rest on the floor. Then push yourself up again. Count how many you can do before growing too tired.

Count the number of squats that you can do to evaluate your lower-body strength. To do a squat, stand up straight with your arms by your sides and legs about shoulder-width apart. Begin to bend your knees as you raise your arms to a horizontal position at your sides. When you have bent your knees so that your thighs are parallel with the ground, go back up again. Then repeat the movement. See how many you can do.

Save these numbers for future comparison. You want to test yourself at intervals of four to six weeks to keep track of your progress and keep yourself motivated to stay on the exercise program.

✔ **Shoulder press:** Stand with your feet shoulder-width apart and knees slightly bent. With dumb-bells in each hand, start with your hands next to your shoulders facing inward. Raise the dumb-bells over your head until your arms are straight. Bring the weights back down to the starting position, palms facing each other.

✔ **Lateral raise:** Hold a dumbbell in each hand by your sides, palms facing each other. Raise the dumbbells out to the sides, keeping your arms straight (but don't lock your elbows) and your palms facing the floor, until they're above your head. Return them to the starting position.

✔ **Bent-over rowing:** Bend from the waist, keeping your knees slightly bent, until your upper body is parallel with the floor. With a dumbbell in each hand and your arms hanging straight down, slowly raise the dumbbells out to the side until they're in line with your shoulders. Lower them again.

✔ **Good mornings:** Stand straight with a single dumbbell held over your head by both hands. Keeping your arms straight over your head, bend from the waist until your torso and arms are parallel with the floor. Then raise yourself to the starting point.

✔ **Flys:** Lie on your back with one dumbbell in each hand and your arms opened out to each side at shoulder height. Slowly raise the dumbbells in over your body until they touch above your chest. Slowly lower them to the starting position.

✔ **Pullovers:** Lie on your back with your knees bent, holding one dumbbell with both hands above your chest. Lower the dumbbell back over your head until it touches the floor. Then raise it back over your chest.

✔ **Curls:** Stand straight up, holding a barbell in each hand in front of you. With your palms facing out, slowly bend your elbows until your hands are shoulder height. Lower them back slowly to the starting position.

A couple of standard exercises for strengthening leg muscles include the following:

- ✔ **Lunges:** Stand straight with your feet about shoulder-width apart. Hold a light dumbbell in each hand, palms facing your body. Take a long step forward with the right foot and bend the right leg until your thigh is parallel with the ground. Hold the position a second, and then step back and straighten your leg. Lunge forward with the other leg.

- ✔ **Squats:** Begin by placing a barbell containing light weights behind your neck, holding it with your hands. Stand straight with your feet hip-width apart. Bend your knees slowly and squat until your thighs are parallel with the ground. Pause, and then rise to the standing position.

You'll be amazed and delighted at the rapid progress you make in terms of body strength, increased fitness, and increased self-assurance if you follow this simple program. Just be sure to increase the weights as they become easier to lift to continue reaping the rewards. Among other benefits, you'll

- ✔ Keep your bones stronger
- ✔ Prevent injuries by improving balance
- ✔ Look better
- ✔ Speed up your metabolism

Using Yoga to lower blood pressure

Yoga is a series of postures and breathing exercises originally developed in India over 5,000 years ago as a way to achieve *union* (yoga) with the "divine consciousness." Today, people often practice Yoga as a way of improving their health and well-being without putting an emphasis on Yoga's religious side. Yoga attempts to unite your body and your mind, so that your mind can function better in a more healthy body.

Numerous studies have shown that Yoga can lower blood pressure. This effect persists as long as the practice continues, and it often disappears if the individual stops practicing Yoga.

An excellent source of information about all aspects of Yoga is *Yoga For Dummies,* by Georg Feuerstein, PhD, and Larry Payne, PhD (Wiley). I highly recommend it to you. The Internet also offers many excellent Yoga sites. The following are two of the best:

- **The Yoga Site** (www.yogasite.com) can answer all your questions and direct you to many other useful sites.

- **The Yoga Directory** (www.yogadirectory.com) directs you to any type of service that you may need that has to do with Yoga from books and publications to centers and organizations, and from retreats and vacations to teachers and training.

Chapter 7

Treating High Blood Pressure with Medications

. . . .

In This Chapter

▶ Getting a grip on drug features and categories

▶ Looking at what drugs expel water, salt, or potassium

▶ Finding the drug that's right for you

▶ Recognizing side effects and brand names

. . . .

*H*ave you done everything in your power to maximize the lifestyle changes that lower the blood pressure without drugs as discussed in Chapters 4 through 6? If you can answer "Yes!" and your blood pressure is still elevated, ask your doctor about giving you a prescription for one of the drugs described in this chapter. If the answer is no, go back and do whatever you can to reduce your blood pressure without drugs.

The choices are limitless, but don't let every cute little new drug that comes along fool you. Designed to manipulate your imagination, glitzy TV and radio commercials and magazine ads suggest that your life can be a bowl of cherries if you pop a new drug. Some drugs are inappropriate for some people with high blood pressure and not others, and some drugs have miserable side effects — side effects that may affect you and just a few other people. Also, if you're already taking another prescription medicine, adding another drug could create a problem.

Your pharmacist can be a great resource for drug information. Also, a publication called the *Physicians' Desk Reference* (PDR) is available in most doctor's offices and hospital libraries. It has the latest information about all drugs.

Presenting the Classes of Drugs

Drugs that lower blood pressure are divided into several different classes, and each class works by a different mechanism. The drugs in this chapter are discussed according to the way that they lower blood pressure. Your doctor may have a preference for one or another drug within a class of drugs.

Many drugs are available in drug combinations, which take advantage of the fact that two drugs of different classes are often more potent together than the sum of each one separately.

Diuretics

Of all the drug classes, the only one that has consistently reduced the illness and death associated with high blood pressure when it's the first treatment is the diuretic class, specifically the thiazide diuretics.

Diuretics, also known as "water pills," lower blood pressure by forcing the body to rid itself of salt and water through the kidneys into the urine. Depending on the place in the kidneys where they're active, diuretics rid the body of more or less salt and water. However, after a couple months, the body overcomes the reduction in body fluids. At this point, it's a reduction in the resistance to blood flow that accounts for the ongoing fall in blood pressure. Diuretics are divided into different groups as follows:

- **Thiazide and thiazidelike diuretic group:** Although they're not the most effective drugs for ridding the body of excess salt and water, the thiazide and thiazidelike diuretic group is the most effective group for lowering blood pressure. This group acts at the nephron, part of the kidney's filtering mechanism to cause the increased excretion of sodium and chloride.

- **Loop diuretics:** The loop diuretics act at the loop of Henle, part of the filtering mechanism of the kidneys. These drugs have a potent effect on salt and water elimination.

- **Potassium-sparing diuretics:** A third group, the potassium-sparing diuretics function at the late distal tubule and the collecting tubule of the nephron. The result is only a mild increase in sodium excretion and chloride excretion but a tendency to reduce the excretion of potassium. Because the other diuretics cause potassium loss, the potassium-sparing diuretics are important for maintaining body potassium.

- **Aldosterone-antagonist group:** This group blocks the action of aldosterone, a natural hormone that causes salt and water retention. If its action is blocked, more salt and water is excreted into the urine while potassium loss is reduced. These drugs could be included in the potassium-sparing group, but they go about lowering blood pressure in an altogether different manner than the potassium-sparing group — they deactivate aldosterone.

Drugs that act on the nervous system

The part of the nervous system that's responsible for increased constriction of the arteries, thus raising blood pressure, is *the sympathetic nervous system.* In 1940, researchers discovered that cutting the nerves of the sympathetic nervous system in the chest and abdomen caused a persistent fall in blood pressure. Since then, scientists have looked for chemical agents that could block the sympathetic nervous system, and they've come up with several. They're broken down into groups by the way they affect the nervous system:

- **Methyldopa** (Aldomet, Methyldopa Tablets) acts within the brain to prevent the release of neurotransmitters so they never get to the receptors. It isn't usually the first drug of choice for high blood pressure because of some rare but serious side effects.

- **Clonidine** (Catapres, Clonidine Hydrochloride Tablets, Clonidine HCl Tablets), guanabenz (Wytensin, Guanabenz Acetate Tablets) and guanfacine (Tenex, Guanfacine Tablets, Guanfacine Hydrochloride Tablets) are similar drugs that lower blood pressure by reducing levels of the chemical messenger norepinephrine that increases blood pressure. They reduce the output of blood from the heart and increase the size of arteries. Because of the sedation that they bring on (and the better characteristics of other drugs), they aren't the drug of choice for treating high blood pressure.

- **Beta-adrenergic receptor blockers,** generally known as beta blockers, are the most important group of drugs that affect the sympathetic nervous system and are second only to the thiazide diuretics in their effectiveness.

Beta blockers aren't the drug of choice for high blood pressure unless the patient has a history of chest pain or heart attack. Beta blockers reduce the forcefulness of the heart while they reduce the secretion of renin and the production of angiotensin II (see Chapter 2). They seem to protect those with atherosclerotic heart disease (see Chapter 3) against pain and further disease.

✔ **Alpha-1 adrenergic receptor antagonists** block another group of sympathetic nerve receptors, some of which are alpha 1 and some alpha 2. Only the alpha-1 blockers are used clinically. Alpha-1 drugs act through different nerve receptors to increase the size of arteries.

Vasodilators

Vasodilators are drugs that relax the muscles in the arteries, making them larger and reducing blood pressure. How this occurs is unclear. If these drugs are given alone, the heart speeds up as the blood pressure falls and patients suffer from headaches, the feeling of a rapid heart beat, and retention of water. Therefore, they're usually given with diuretics to get rid of water and beta blockers to slow the heart.

Doctors use two vasodilators, hydralazine and minoxidil, usually for the most difficult cases because of their side effects. Those side effects are as follows:

✔ Hydralazine's side effects include headaches, nausea, excess reduction in blood pressure, feeling of a rapid heartbeat, dizziness, and heart pain if there is coronary artery disease. Interestingly, although hydralazine expands some arteries of the heart, it doesn't expand certain other arteries in the heart. The result is that blood is "stolen" from one area to another. The area that loses blood may develop pain.

Hydralazine also causes retention of water and can result in heart failure, so it's usually given with both a diuretic and a beta blocker.

Hydralazine also causes the occurrence of an allergic reaction against the body's own tissues called the *lupus syndrome.* This begins only after at least six months of treatment and is more frequent as the dose goes higher. After the drug is stopped, the condition usually subsides.

✔ Minoxidil causes salt and water retention, increased heart rate and strength of heart contractions, and increased hair growth on the face, back, arms, and legs.

Calcium channel blocking agents

Calcium channel blocking agents (also known as calcium channel blockers) take advantage of the fact that in order for a muscle in an artery to contract to make the artery smaller, calcium has to move into the muscle cell. These agents block that movement, and the muscle relaxes, resulting in larger arteries and lower blood pressure.

As arteries widen and peripheral resistance declines, the body responds by increasing the heart rate. This isn't true of all calcium channel blocking agents, however. Certain calcium channel blocking agents, particularly verapamil, nifedipine, and diltiazem, slow the heart, so the heart rate doesn't increase when these are used.

Calcium channel blockers aren't the first or second drug of choice for blood pressure treatment among people with enlarged hearts or heart failure. Calcium channel blockers also shouldn't be the first or second choice of treatment for high blood pressure after a heart attack. They decrease muscle contraction, an undesirable effect when the heart is already failing or weakened by a heart attack.

When heart disease doesn't already exist, calcium channel blockers can lower blood pressure as effectively as beta blockers. When a heart attack has occurred, calcium channel blockers don't improve survival the way that beta blockers do.

These drugs have several side effects, but these side effects rarely cause the patient to stop taking the drug. The main side effects are headache, flushing in the face, dizziness, and swelling of the legs. To overcome these side effects, sustained-release preparations have been developed.

These agents are safe in the presence of diabetes, asthma, kidney abnormalities, and when blood fats are abnormal. So calcium channel blockers can be useful, even though they're not the first choice for treating high blood pressure.

A number of calcium channel blockers are available and are classified by their chemical structure. One group that does not have the same underlying chemical structure, consists of verapamil and diltiazem. The second group, all connected by having a similar chemical structure, consist of amlodipine, felodipine, asradipine, nicardipine, nifedipine and nisoldipine, all of which end in "pine."

Angiotensin-converting enzyme inhibitors

Angiotensin-converting enzyme (ACE) *inhibitors* affect the activity of the renin-angiotensin-aldosterone system, which helps the kidney moderate blood pressure. Angiotension-converting enzyme converts a hormone called angiotensin I to angiotensin II. Angiotensin II raises blood pressure two ways: It causes direct contraction of arteries, and it causes the adrenal gland to release aldosterone (see Chapter 2), which, in turn, causes salt and water retention.

The ACE inhibitors block the angiotensin-converting enzyme so that angiotensin II isn't made. ACE inhibitors can make thiazide diuretics more effective by blocking the tendency of the body to make more aldosterone as water and salt are lost.

While it prevents the increase in blood pressure, the ACE inhibitor also leads to a fall in blood pressure because angiotensin II also breaks down *bradykinen,* a hormone that causes widening of blood vessels. In the absence of angiotensin II, *bradykinen* levels are increased.

This class of drugs is especially important for people with heart failure, kidney disease, diabetes, and other kidney problems. More than any other drug for high blood pressure, ACE inhibitors slow the progression of these diseases, so they're especially useful when these conditions are present.

One advantage of the ACE inhibitors is that they don't cause changes in blood fats, blood sugar, and uric acid, or a fall in potassium. Another major advantage of the ACE inhibitors is the low number of side effects. Potential side effects include the following:

✔ Elevations in serum potassium levels, especially in patients with heart failure or reduced kidney function

✔ Abnormally low blood pressure if the patient has decreased blood volume to begin with as, for example, after treatment with a diuretic

> ✔ A dry cough, which occurs in 20 percent of patients who receive the drug

Rare side effects include a rash, loss of taste, and reduction of white blood cells.

A very rare but potentially fatal complication is *angioneurotic edema,* which causes the throat to swell severely and make breathing troubled. These drugs should be stopped immediately if such signs and symptoms develop.

An ACE inhibitor paired with a potassium-sparing diuretic or spironolactone can be dangerous because both cause increase blood potassium.

ACE inhibitors should absolutely not be used during pregnancy or in a young woman who plans to become pregnant soon because they've been known to damage the growing fetus. Likewise, they shouldn't be used during breast-feeding to avoid damage to the nursing infant.

When ACE inhibitors are compared with diuretics, beta blockers, and calcium channel blockers, they don't lower blood pressure as effectively as these other drugs. When compared in terms of decreasing sickness and death, ACE inhibitors aren't as effective as diuretics or beta blockers but better than calcium channel blockers.

Numerous ACE inhibitors are available with some variation in their breakdown. They can be recognized by the fact that their names end in "pril."

Angiotensin II receptor blockers

These drugs, rather than blocking the enzyme as the ACE inhibitors do, block angiotensin II by not allowing it to attach to its receptor where it does its work of

contracting arteries and releasing aldosterone.
Because angiotensin II can be made by other enzymes
besides angiotensin-converting enzyme, inhibition of
angiotensin II by ACE inhibitors isn't complete.
These receptor blockers can eliminate the activity of
angiotensin II more completely. Drugs in this group all
end with "artan."

Like the ACE inhibitors, these drugs are similar to one
another. They have the advantage over ACE inhibitors
in that they don't cause the dry cough. Recent studies
of irbesartan and losartan show that they effectively
reverse kidney disease in diabetes. This occurred
even when the drug didn't lower the blood pressure
much.

They're relatively free of side effects although they
can cause elevation in potassium because they're
similar to the ACE inhibitors in their action.
Occasional patients (less than 1 percent of those who
take these drugs) develop headache or dizziness and
have to discontinue the drugs. A rare patient develops
facial swelling. Drug interactions don't seem to be a
problem with this class.

These drugs don't change blood-fat levels, increase
the uric acid, or increase the sugar in the blood. They
are metabolized in the body into inactive substances,
so elimination doesn't depend on the liver or the
kidneys.

Like the ACE inhibitors, angiotensin II receptor
blockers shouldn't be prescribed for pregnant
or breast-feeding women. Nor should they be
prescribed for young women who plan to
become pregnant soon.

Choosing a Drug

Now that you know all about the drugs that you can take to control your blood pressure, you're ready to put that information to use. Sure, your doctor makes the decisions about which medication to use, but you have the right to have some input, because that drug goes into *your* body, not your doctor's.

Treating uncomplicated high blood pressure

Some basic principles that doctors use for starting treatment follow:

- Ideally, use a drug that can be given once a day, that's cheap, and has few side effects.

- Start with a very low dose, maybe half the recommended dose; this is especially important for the elderly.

- Increase the dose slowly until the desired effect is reached.

- If the pressure isn't controlled at a reasonable dose, add a second drug with a different mechanism of action, or switch to another drug with a different mechanism of action. Again, start at a low dose and build up gradually.

- If the drug isn't tolerated because of side effects, discontinue it, and try a drug with a different mechanism of action.

This assumes that you don't have heart failure, eye disease, kidney disease, heart attacks, or other complications.

Start with a diuretic, preferably hydrochlorothiazide, at a low dose of 12.5 or 25 mg daily. Give this at least two months to lower your blood pressure while getting your potassium checked occasionally. If the potassium falls abnormally low, add a potassium-sparing agent, probably amiloride.

Because higher doses don't seem to lower the blood pressure any better than low doses of hydrochlorothiazide, the next step, if necessary, is the addition of a beta-blocking drug. The one that has proven itself in clinical trials is propranolol. It's given in a starting dose of 20 mg twice daily. Some physicians recommend starting with a drug combination, such as Propranolol Hydrochloride and Hydrochlorothiazide tablets and not bothering to use one drug. If the blood pressure is only mildly elevated, this isn't necessary.

Treating complicated high blood pressure

A number of different complications cause your choice to move away from the diuretics to some drug that can manage both the high blood pressure and the complication. The most important of these are as follows:

✔ Heart failure is best treated by an ACE inhibitor and a diuretic. The diuretic in this case may not be one of the thiazide diuretics but the more powerful loop diuretics because too much fluid in the body is one of the major problems.

✔ Chest pain due to disease in the coronary arteries along with high blood pressure does better with beta blockers or calcium channel blockers.

✔ A heart attack with high blood pressure responds better to a beta blocker and an ACE inhibitor as the first choice. Although diltiazem and verapamil, calcium channel blockers, have shown the ability to reduce sickness and death in this situation.

✔ Diabetes mellitus with kidney disease and high blood pressure is best managed by an ACE inhibitor or one of the angiotensin II receptor blockers.

✔ Heart rhythm abnormalities with high blood pressure do better on beta blockers or calcium channel blockers, such as verapamil or diltiazem, but not nifedipine.

✔ Fat abnormalities in the blood along with high blood pressure are better treated with beta blockers that don't cause further fat abnormalities.

✔ Hand tremors along with high blood pressure may respond better to certain beta blockers, such as propranolol.

✔ If hyperthyroidism is present in addition to high blood pressure, a beta blocker is definitely the drug of choice.

✔ People with migraine headaches and high blood pressure do better with certain beta blockers or calcium channel blockers, such as propranolol or diltiazem.

✔ A person about to undergo surgery who has high blood pressure does better if the blood pressure medication during the surgery is a beta blocker.

When the first choice fails

If a prescription can't keep the blood pressure consistently under 140/90 mm Hg, further action must be taken. If it's because the blood pressure doesn't respond or the side effects are intolerable, a drug from another class is given. If the diuretics and beta blockers can't be used, the next step is an ACE inhibitor.

If the blood pressure is only partially controlled, a second drug from another drug class is added. If a diuretic hasn't been added, it should be added at this point. Then if the blood pressure still doesn't get down under 140/90 mm Hg, a third drug is added.

You should see your doctor again within one month after a change in medication.

Just because it took several drugs to bring your blood pressure under control doesn't necessarily mean that you're going to take all these drugs for the rest of your life. If you can lose weight or use some other method to bring down your blood pressure without drugs, you may be able to reduce dosages or stop some of the drugs. Even without other improvements, after a year of control, trying to cut down on some of the drugs under the care of your doctor is worthwhile.

Recognizing Drug Side Effects

None of the drugs listed in this chapter is perfect; they all cause side effects and some of them are so severe that the drug must be discontinued. Being aware of side effects is important. If you notice an uncomfortable change shortly after you start a new drug for high blood pressure, it's relatively easy to know that the drug is to blame. Sometimes the side effect doesn't become apparent until months after you start the drug. At other times, the addition of another drug, often one that's used to treat another disease, brings out the side effect of the first drug.

 If something in the list of side effects describes how you're feeling, discuss it with your doctor and consider a reduction in dosage or a change in the medication to a different class of drugs.

 Drugs in the same class usually have the same side effects. To rid yourself of an annoying side effect, you have to switch to a new class.

Side Effect	*Drug That May Cause It*
Anemia	Methyldopa
Breast enlargement	Spironolactone
Confusion	All diuretics
Constipation	Calcium channel blockers
Decreased good cholesterol	Beta blockers
Decreased white blood cells	ACE inhibitors
Depression	Clonidine, guanabenz, guanfacine, and calcium channel blockers
Diarrhea	Potassium-sparing diuretics
Dizziness	All diuretics, labetalol, and doxazocin
Dry cough	ACE inhibitors
Dry eyes	Clonidine, guanabenz, and guanfacine
Dry mouth	All diuretics, methyldopa, clonidine, guanabenz, and guanfacine
Fatigue	Beta blockers and doxazocin

Fever	Methyldopa, labetalol
Fluid in breasts	Methyldopa
Headache	Vasodilators and calcium channel blockers
Heart failure	Alpha-1 adrenergic receptor antagonists and vasodilators
Increased asthma	Beta blockers
Increased blood sugar	All diuretics
Increased cholesterol	Thiazide diuretics
Increased hairiness	Spironolactone and minoxidil
Increased urination	All diuretics
Irritation of the esophagus	Calcium channel blockers
Liver damage	Methyldopa
Loss of hearing	Loop diuretics
Loss of taste	ACE inhibitors
Lupus syndrome	Hydralazine
Menstrual irregularities	Spironolactone
Muscle pains	All diuretics
Nausea and vomiting	All diuretics
Rapid heart beat	Vasodilators
Reduced erections	Thiazide diuretics, spironolactone, and methyldopa
Skin rashes	All diuretics
Sleepiness	Methyldopa, clonidine, guanabenz, and guanfacine
Swelling of the abdomen	Potassium-sparing diuretics
Swelling of the legs	Vasodilators

Thirst	All diuretics
Very low blood pressure	ACE inhibitors
Vivid dreams or nightmares	Clonidine, guanabenz, and guanfacine
Weakness	All diuretics

These are the most common side effects identified with the drugs for high blood pressure. Many more less common problems aren't listed. If you have an unusual new symptom after starting a drug, by all means, discuss it with your doctor and consider a reduction in dose or a change in medication.

Identifying Brand Names

So many drugs, so many brand names. How can you know what you're on, much less what it does and what its side effects may be?

In this section, I provide all the brand names of the current drugs in alphabetical order. Look up the brand name, and then refer to the drug's scientific name in the right column to find out what you're taking. You may discover that you're on a drug that you would be better off without, or it may explain that irritating symptom you've been having.

Always keep an up-to-date list of all of your drugs, preferably by scientific and brand name. You should have the milligrams of the pill and the amount and frequency with which you take it. It can save your doctor plenty of time when prescription renewals are needed and any new doctor you see will know more about your health by the drugs you're taking.

Some of these drugs are no longer made under
their brand name because the patent has run
out, and competing against a generic form of the
drug is no longer profitable for the drug company. However, the doctor may still be using the
brand name because he has always called it by
that name, so you'll need to know the brand
name anyway.

Brand Name	*Scientific Name*
Accupril	Quinapril
Accuretic	Quinapril and hydrochlorothiazide
Aceon	Perinopril
Adalat	Nifedipine
Aldactone	Spironolactone
Aldactazide	Spironolactone and hydrochlorothiazide
Aldoclor	Methyldopa and chlorothiazide
Aldomet	Methyldopa
Aldoril	Methyldopa and hydrochlorothiazide
Altace	Ramipril
Apresoline	Hydralazine
Apresozide	Hydralazine and hydrochlorothiazide
Aquatensen	Methyclorthiazide
Atacand	Candesartan cilexitil
Avalide	Irbesartan and hydrochlorothiazide
Avapro	Irbesartan
Blocardren	Timolol
Bumex	Bumetanide
Calan	Verapamil

Capoten	Captopril
Capozide	Captopril and hydrochlorothiazide
Cardizem CD	Diltiazem
Cardura	Doxazosin
Cartrol Filmtab Tablets	Carteolol
Catapres	Clonidine
Clorpres	Clonidine and chlorthalidone
Combipres	Clonidine and chlorthalidone
Coreg	Carvedilol
Corzide	Nadolol and bendroflumethiazide
Covera	Verapamil
Cozaar	Losartan
Demadex	Torsemide
Dilicor XR	Diltiazem
Diovan	Valsartan
Diovan HCT	Valsartan and hydrochlorothiazide
Diuril Oral Suspension	Chlorothiazide
Diuril Tablets	Chlorothiazide
Dyazide	Triamterene and hydrochlorothiazide
Dyrenium	Triamterene
Edecrin	Ethacrynic acid
Enduron Tablets	Methyclorthiazide
HydroDIURIL	Hydrochlorothiazide
Hygroton	Chlorthalidone
Hytrin	Terzosin
Hyzaar	Losartan and hydrochlorothiazide
Inderal	Propranolol

Inderide	Propranolol and hydrochlorothiazide
Isoptin	Verapamil
Lasix	Furosemide
Levatol	Penbutolol
Lexxel	Felodipine and enalapril
Loniten	Minoxidil
Lopressor	Metoprolol
Lotensin	Benazepril
Lotrel	Amlodipine and benazepril
Lozol	Indapamide
Mavik	Trandolapril
Maxide	Triamterene and hydrochlorothiazide
Midamor	Amiloride
Minipress	Prazosin
Minizide	Prazosin and polyzide
Miscardis	Telmisartan
Moduretic	Amiloride and hydrochlorothiazide
Monopril	Fosinopril
Mykrox	Metolazone
Naturetin	Bendroflumethiazide
Normodyne	Labetalol
Norvasc	Amlodipine
Oretic	Hydrochlorothiazide
Plendil	Felodipine
Prinivil	Lisinopril
Prinzide	Lisinopril and hydrochlorothiazide
Procardia	Nifedipine
Renese	Polythiazide
Sectral	Acebutolol

Sular	Nisoldipine
Tarka	Trandolapril and verapamil
Teczem	Diltiazem and enalapril
Tenex	Guanfacine
Tenormine	Atenolol
Teveten	Eprosartan
Thalitone	Chlorthalidone
Tiazac	Diltiazem
Timolide	Timolol and hydrochlorothiazide
Toprol XL	Metoprolol
Trandate	Labetalol
Uniretic	Moexipril and hydrochlorothiazide
Univasc	Moexipril
Vasotec	Enalapril
Verelan	Verapamil
Wytensin	Guanabenz
Zaroxolyn	Metolazone
Zebeta	Bisoprolol
Zestril	Lisinopril
Zestoretic	Lisinopril and hydrochlorothiazide
Ziac	Bisoprolol and hydrochlorothiazide

Chapter 8

Ten Myths about High Blood Pressure

....

In This Chapter

▶ Investigating misunderstandings about high blood pressure

▶ Discovering the realities of high blood pressure

....

*M*yths about high blood pressure are numerous, and selecting only ten is difficult. I tried to pick out the myths that have the most impact on your high blood pressure. My hope is that after you have your misunderstandings cleared up by this chapter, you'll take many or all of the actions described in this book and take complete control of your blood pressure.

You Can Skip Your Medication When You're Feeling Fine

High blood pressure is sometimes called the "silent killer." People are often unaware that they have high blood pressure. It can do damage to the eyes, heart, kidneys, and blood vessels, but symptoms don't appear until an organ begins to fail. When the organ begins to fail, it's too late to reverse the damage.

A lack of symptoms is the reason that many people neglect to take their blood pressure medication. They felt fine before they started taking the pills. The only reason they're taking the pills is because their doctor measured a high blood pressure. In fact, as a result of the side effects of the pills, they may feel worse when taking the pills.

Not taking your blood pressure medication isn't a good idea. The point of taking the medication is to lower your pressure and in turn, to prevent complications, such as heart attacks and brain attacks. These complications probably take ten years or more to develop. Bringing your blood pressure down into the normal range through lifestyle changes and medication if necessary gives you time to steer clear of these complications.

If side effects from the medication are a problem, discuss the possibility of lowering the dose or switching to another medicine with your doctor.

Medications can help you control your blood pressure and avoid the serious damage, or even death, that high blood pressure causes. Don't fail to make use of them.

You Need Treatment Only for a High Diastolic Blood Pressure

Treating a high diastolic blood pressure only was once the way that blood pressure control was practiced, and it hasn't disappeared from the treatment plan of many doctors. But you know better.

Both the diastolic blood pressure and the systolic blood pressure figure in the decision to lower blood pressure. The goal is to maintain a number under 140 for the systolic blood pressure and a number under 90 for the diastolic blood pressure.

Diastolic blood pressure tends to fall with age while systolic blood pressure tends to rise. For example, studies show that people under the age of 50 who have high blood pressure usually have diastolic high blood pressure. The much larger group of people over the age of 50 who have high blood pressure usually has isolated systolic high blood pressure. According to these numbers, if treatment were based on the diastolic blood pressure alone, very few people would receive treatment for high blood pressure detected after the age of 50. Yet treating people over age 50 for high blood pressure greatly reduces the number of heart attacks and brain attacks in this age group.

High Blood Pressure Can't Be Controlled

If you're diagnosed with high blood pressure and take your medication regularly, but your blood pressure doesn't come down into the acceptable range of 140/90 mm Hg, don't give up — and definitely don't stop taking your medication. Instead, with the help of your doctor, take another look at your medication and lifestyle to see whether you can do more to control your blood pressure. Rest assured, an explanation for your inability to bring your blood pressure under control can be found. The means to control high blood pressure in all patients currently exist. It's up to you and your doctor to find the right solution.

Start by making sure that your blood pressure is uncontrolled. Could it be a case of faulty measurement? Is your blood pressure normal except when you step into the doctor's office (white coat effect)? You may have to get your own blood pressure device and check it for yourself at home.

Take a closer look at your medication. Resistance to treatment is defined as the inability of a combination of three different types of medications from three different classes, one of which is a diuretic, to lower the blood pressure to less than 140/90 mm Hg.

Are you maximizing your use of lifestyle changes to squeeze every millimeter of mercury out of those procedures? You can't say that your blood pressure can't be controlled until you have tried all of the lifestyle measures that doctors know can lower blood pressure.

Discuss the possibility that you have secondary high blood pressure (see Chapter 2) with your doctor. The diseases and conditions that can cause second high blood pressure, such as blocked kidney arteries or a tumor in an adrenal gland, are rare but may account for the stubborn resistance of your blood pressure to treatment.

The Treatment Is Worse Than the Disease

The consequences of untreated high blood pressure at any age are far greater than the side effects of medication or the inconveniences of lifestyle changes. To begin with, use nondrug treatments, such as lowering your salt and caffeine intake and exercising regularly, to their fullest extent. (See Chapters 4 through 6 for more ways that you can adjust your lifestyle to lower your blood pressure.)

Many of the nondrug treatments not only lower your blood pressure but also provide you with all kinds of other benefits. The peacefulness that comes from exercising, yoga, and meditation can't be found in any blood pressure medicine.

If your doctor determines that your blood pressure should be treated with medication, don't have a crisis. Sure, blood pressure medications have side effects, and you'll probably feel better without them. But there aren't too many side effects that are worse than the effects of untreated high blood pressure — namely heart attacks, brain attacks, and kidney failure.

 The side effects can be overcome in several ways. Work with your doctor to determine the combination of lifestyle changes and medications that's right for you.

Only Nervous, Anxious People Get High Blood Pressure

A high level of nervousness and anxiety doesn't indicate that a person has or will have high blood pressure. A nervous, anxious person may have normal blood pressure, while a person who appears quite calm and peaceful may have exceedingly high blood pressure.

This myth probably developed from the short name for high blood pressure — hypertension. The prefix *hyper* suggests that sufferers are highly stressed, jumpy, and nervous individuals, who live a life of anger and road rage and have a short fuse, making them ready to blow up at any moment. The suffix *tension* certainly doesn't suggest a calm, peaceful state of being. However, that people with high blood pressure come only from this group isn't the case.

People with high blood pressure are found in every social class, doing every type of work. And although high blood pressure tends to be a disease of the overweight, it's certainly found among thin people. People with high blood pressure aren't necessarily type A overachievers working 14-hour days. It would certainly make doctors' diagnostic abilities much better if they could pick out people who have high blood pressure from one group with certain personality traits, but it doesn't work that way.

You Can't Exercise If You Have High Blood Pressure

This myth provides an excuse for many people who don't want to exercise. It's totally and unequivocally false. And exercise lowers blood pressure.

How did this myth get started? It probably began when some people with severe, uncontrolled high blood pressure and major complications of the condition did some exercise and got into trouble. If you have unstable heart disease associated with high blood pressure, for example, you can have a heart attack as a result of heavy exercise.

If you have heart disease or if you have had a heart attack or a brain attack, ask your physician what exercises you can do safely. You may find that there are no limitations. Or you may find that it's safer for you to avoid certain activities that are too vigorous or require too much effort over a short period of time, such as heavy weight lifting. But there's no reason for you to avoid physical activity if your high blood pressure is under control.

If you have high blood pressure and no complications, the benefits of exercise are enormous. You don't have to run marathons or do triathlons. One half hour of walking a day provides great benefits.

The old adage for physical exercise used to be, "No pain, no gain." The new one is, "Refrain, no gain."

The Elderly Don't Need to Treat Their High Blood Pressure

Some people believe that it's too late or not helpful to treat high blood pressure in the elderly. High blood pressure is most prevalent in the elderly population, the people that I have arbitrarily selected as age 75 or older. They're also the people who have the highest number of heart attacks and brain attacks each year. If they get treatment for their high blood pressure, large numbers of these attacks can be prevented. If they're not treated, some of them die earlier than they might normally have, and some of them will be subjected to years of disability.

You Have to Restrict Your Life Because of High Blood Pressure

Although high blood pressure is a serious condition that must be managed with lifestyle change and drugs if necessary, restricting your life isn't reasonable. You should be able to live a normal life within the limitations of any side effects caused by the drugs that you're taking.

If you have uncomplicated high blood pressure, you should have about the same quality of life as a person with normal blood pressure. Your quality of life can be even better because you're taking better care of your body. You may consider limiting salt intake and kilocalories as a restriction on your life and to some extent they are. On the other hand, they could be looked upon as enhancing the quality of your life. Taking salt out of your diet gives you a chance to taste some amazing foods that were hidden behind the strong taste of salt. Restricting kilocalories and losing some weight makes you feel better about yourself, more attractive, and healthier.

Stopping Treatment after a Heart or Brain Attack Is Okay

You shouldn't stop treating high blood pressure after you recover from a heart or brain attack. The risks of complications from high blood pressure are great after a heart or brain attack; therefore, controlling your blood pressure after one of these attacks is important. One of the main risk factors for a heart attack or a brain attack is a previous heart or brain attack. You need to make sure that your blood pressure is kept under control more than ever.

The changes that you make to control your high blood pressure can help your diabetes and your arthritis, as well as your heart and blood vessels.

High Blood Pressure Is Less Dangerous in Women

The consequences of high blood pressure for women are as serious as those for men. Blood pressure control is just as important for women as it is for men.

Although three out of four women who have high blood pressure are aware of it, only one of those three has her high blood pressure under control. In other words, 75 percent of women with high blood pressure don't control it. This is a tragic situation for many women with high blood pressure.

The extremely dangerous disorders called *preeclampsia* and *eclampsia* that can begin in the 20th week of a pregnancy are ignored only at great risk to the mother and the growing fetus.

Estrogen may play an important role in women who are postmenopausal with high blood pressure. Estrogen replacement therapy can lower blood pressure in these women by as much as 10/5 mm Hg.

Even at the other end of the age spectrum, women in their 70s and 80s represent a large proportion of the high blood pressure among all people at that age. Fifty percent of all white women and 80 percent of all black women in the United States over age 60 have high blood pressure. These women suffer heart attacks and brain attacks at a much higher rate when their high blood pressure isn't controlled.

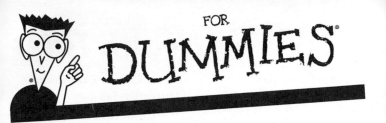

FOR DUMMIES®

What makes **For Dummies** *Health titles so popular?*

Whenever a condition is diagnosed, people need fast, easy-to-understand answers.

Readers get the essential information on treatments, medications, and lifestyle changes. They'll also find out how to begin and maintain an exercise program and stick to healthy eating habits.

Our health titles feature:
- Expert authors with excellent credentials. In fact – many of our authors still work daily in the medical profession
- Content that can be used by both the patient and caregiver
- Local editions where applicable
- A comprehensive approach to treating or managing the condition – from medications to diet and exercise

DUMMIES FOR *Health Titles*

Acne For Dummies
978-0-471-74698-0 • 312 pp.
$16.99 US • $21.99 CAN • £11.99 UK

AD/HD For Dummies
978-0-7645-3712-7 • 356 pp.
$19.99 US • $25.99 CAN • £13.99 UK

Alzheimer's For Dummies
978-0-7645-3899-5 • 384 pp.
$21.99 US • $31.99 CAN • £14.99 UK

**Arthritis For Dummies,
2nd Edition**
978-0-7645-7074-2 • 380 pp.
$19.99 US • $25.99 CAN • £13.99 UK

**Arthritis For Dummies,
UK Edition**
978-0-470-02582-6 • 400 pp.
£14.99 UK

Asthma For Dummies
978-0-7645-4233-6 • 380 pp.
$19.99 US • $25.99 CAN • £12.99 UK

**Asthma & Allergies For
Dummies, Australian Edition**
978-1-74031-054-3 • 272 pp.
$39.95 AUS

**Back Pain Remedies For
Dummies**
978-0-7645-5132-1 • 384 pp.
$19.99 US • $25.99 CAN • £14.99 UK

Breast Cancer For Dummies
978-0-7645-2482-0 • 384 pp.
$21.99 US • $28.99 CAN • £15.50 UK

**Breast Cancer For Dummies,
Australian Edition**
978-1-74031-143-4 • 376 pp.
$39.95 AUS

**The Calorie Counter For
Dummies**
978-0-470-56834-7 • 448 pp.
$7.99 US • $9.99 CAN • £5.99 UK

**The Calorie Counter Journal
For Dummies**
978-0-470-63998-6 • 448 pp.
$12.99 US • £12.99 UK

Celiac Disease For Dummies
978-0-470-16036-7 • 384 pp.
$19.99 US • $23.99 CAN

**Chemotherapy and
Radiation For Dummies**
978-0-7645-7832-8 • 380 pp.
$21.99 US • $28.99 CAN • £13.99 UK

**Chronic Fatigue Syndrome
For Dummies**
978-0-470-11772-9 • 384 pp.
$21.99 US • $25.99 CAN • £14.99 UK

Chronic Pain For Dummies
978-0-471-75140-3 • 384 pp.
$19.99 US • $25.99 CAN • £13.99 UK

**Complementary Medicine
For Dummies, UK Edition**
978-0-470-02625-0 • 448 pp.
£15.99 UK

DUMMIES *Health Titles*

Conquering Childhood Obesity For Dummies
978-0-471-79146-1 • 338 pp.
$19.99 US • $25.99 CAN • £13.99 UK

Controlling Cholesterol For Dummies
978-0-7645-5440-7 • 360 pp.
$21.99 US • $28.99 CAN • £16.50 UK

COPD For Dummies
978-0-470-24757-0 • 338 pp.
$19.99 US • $21.99 CAN • £13.99 UK

Cosmetic Surgery For Dummies
978-0-7645-7835-9 • 382 pp.
$21.99 US • $30.99 CAN • £14.99 UK

Diabetes Cookbook For Dummies, 3rd Edition
978-0-470-53644-5 • 392 pp.
$19.99 US • $23.99 CAN

Diabetes Cookbook For Dummies, UK Edition
978-0-470-51219-7 • 384 pp.
£15.99 UK

Diabetes For Canadians For Dummies, 2nd Edition
978-0-470-15677-3 • 408 pp.
$29.99 CAN

Diabetes For Dummies, 3rd Edition
978-0-470-27086-8 • 408 pp.
$21.99 US

Diabetes For Dummies, 2nd Australian Edition
978-1-74031-094-9 • 544 pp.
$39.95 AUS

Diabetes For Dummies, 2nd UK Edition
978-0-470-05810-7 • 396 pp.
£15.99 UK

Eating Disorders For Dummies
978-0-470-22549-3 • 364 pp.
$19.99 US • $21.99 CAN • £13.99 UK

Endometriosis For Dummies
978-0-470-05047-7 • 362 pp.
$21.99 US • $25.99 CAN • £14.99 UK

Fertility & Infertility For Dummies, UK Edition
978-0-470-05750-6 • 384 pp.
£15.99 UK

Fibromyalgia For Dummies, 2nd Edition
978-0-470-14502-9 • 360 pp.
$21.99 US • $28.99 CAN • £16.50 UK

Food Allergies For Dummies
978-0-470-09584-3 • 384 pp.
$19.99 US • $23.99 CAN • £13.99 UK

Gluten-Free Cooking For Dummies
978-0-470-17810-2 • 342 pp.
$19.99 US • $21.99 CAN • £13.99 UK

DUMMIES *Health Titles*

The Glycemic Index Diet For Dummies
978-0-470-53870-8 • 384 pp.
$19.99 US • $23.99 CAN • £14.99 UK

Hair Loss & Replacement For Dummies
978-0-470-08787-9 • 336 pp.
$16.99 US • $18.99 CAN • £11.99 UK

Healing Foods For Dummies
978-0-7645-5198-7 • 352 pp.
$19.99 US • $27.99 CAN • £14.99 UK

Healthy Aging For Dummies
978-0-470-14975-1 • 384 pp.
$21.99 US • $25.99 CAN • £14.99 UK

The Healthy Heart Cookbook For Dummies
978-0-7645-5222-9 • 384 pp.
$19.99 US • $27.99 CAN • £14.99 UK

Heart Disease For Dummies
978-0-7645-4155-1 • 384 pp.
$19.99 US • $23.99 CAN • £12.99 UK

Heartburn & Reflux For Dummies
978-0-7645-5688-3 • 360 pp.
$19.99 US • $25.99 CAN • £13.99 UK

Herbal Remedies For Dummies
978-0-7645-5127-7 • 384 pp.
$21.99 US • $25.99 CAN • £16.50 UK

High Blood Pressure For Dummies, 2nd Edition
978-0-470-13751-2 • 360 pp.
$21.99 US • $25.99 CAN • £16.50 UK

Hypoglycemia For Dummies, 2nd Edition
978-0-470-12170-2 • 288 pp.
$16.99 US • $21.99 CAN • £12.95 UK

IBS Cookbook For Dummies
978-0-470-53072-6 • 360 pp.
$21.99 US • $25.99 CAN • £15.99 UK

IBS For Dummies
978-0-7645-9814-2 • 384 pp.
$19.99 US • $23.99 CAN • £12.99 UK

IBS For Dummies, UK Edition
978-0-470-51737-6 • 402 pp.
£15.99 UK

Infertility For Dummies
978-0-470-11518-3 • 362 pp.
$21.99 US • $25.99 CAN

Living Dairy-Free For Dummies
978-0-470-63316-8 • 384 pp.
$19.99 US • $23.99 CAN • £14.99 UK

Living Gluten-Free For Dummies, 2nd Edition
978-0-470-58589-4 • 384 pp.
$19.99 US • $23.99 CAN

DUMMIES *Health Titles*

Living Gluten-free For Dummies, Australian Edition
978-0-731-40760-6 • 200 pp.
$34.95 AUS

Living Gluten Free For Dummies, UK Edition
978-0-470-31910-9 • 384 pp.
£15.99 UK

Living With Hepatitis C For Dummies
978-0-7645-7620-1 • 312 pp.
$16.99 US • $19.99 CAN • £11.99 UK

Low-Cholesterol Cookbook For Dummies
978-0-7645-7160-2 • 384 pp.
$19.99 US • $25.99 CAN

Low-Cholesterol Cookbook For Dummies, UK Edition
978-0-470-71401-0 • 384 pp.
£15.99 UK

Macrobiotics For Dummies
978-0-470-40138-5 • 384 pp.
$19.99 US •$21.99 CAN • £13.99 UK

Managing PCOS For Dummies, UK Edition
978-0-470-05794-0 • 376 pp.
£15.99 UK

Medical Ethics For Dummies
978-0-470-87856-9• 384 pp.
$24.99 US • $29.99 CAN • £17.99 UK

Medical Terminology For Dummies
978-0-470-27965-6 • 384 pp.
$21.99 US • $23.99 CAN • £14.99 UK

Medicare Prescription Drugs For Dummies
978-0-470-27676-1 • 384 pp.
$19.99 US • $21.99 CAN • £10.99 UK

Menopause For Dummies, 2nd Edition
978-0-470-05343-0 • 384 pp.
$21.99 US • $25.99 CAN

Menopause For Dummies, Australian Edition
978-1-74031-140-3 • 363 pp.
$39.95 AUS

Menopause For Dummies, UK Edition
978-0-470-06100-8 • 384 pp.
£15.99 UK

Migraines For Dummies
978-0-7645-5485-8 • 330 pp.
$19.99 US • $25.99 CAN • £14.95 UK

Multiple Sclerosis For Dummies
978-0-470-05592-2 • 362 pp.
$21.99 US • $25.99 CAN • £14.99 UK

Obsessive Compulsive Disorder For Dummies
978-0-47029331-7 • 384 pp.
$19.99 US • $21.99 CAN • £13.99 UK

DUMMIES^{FOR} *Health Titles*